Contents

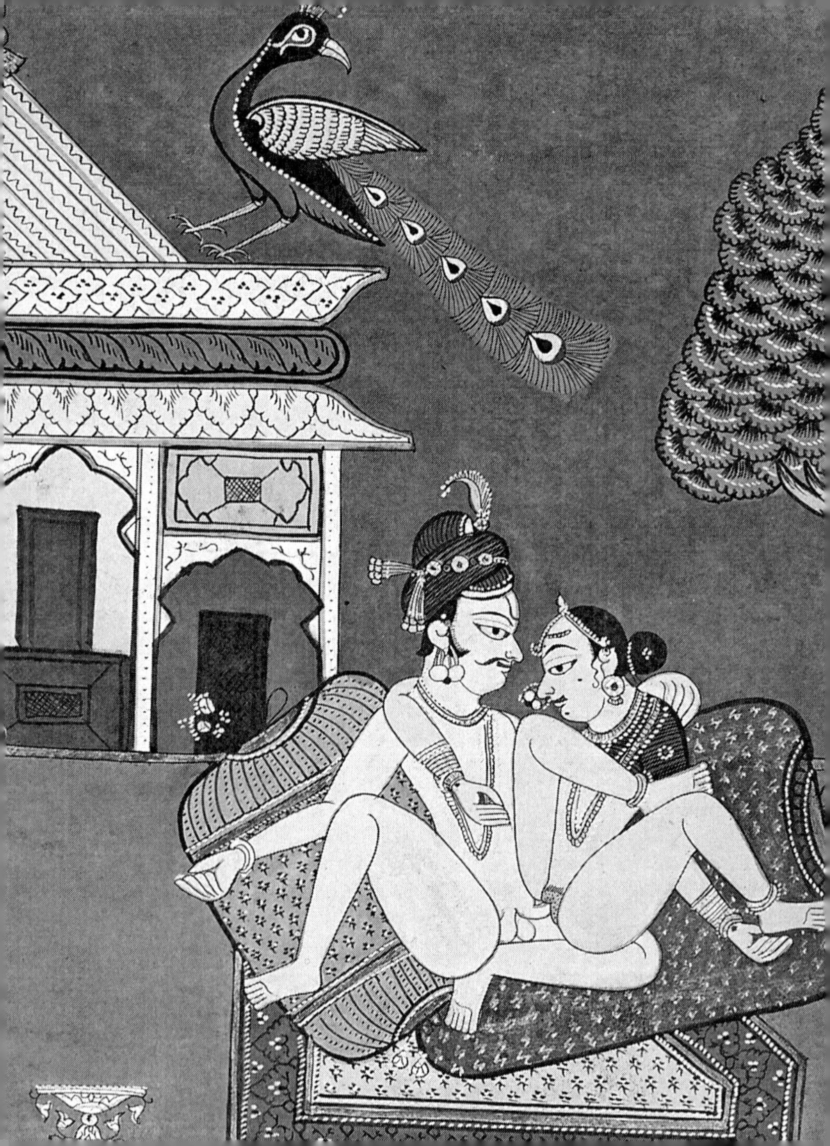

Introduction

'Dharma is better than Artha, and Artha is better than Kama. But Artha should always be first practised by the king, for the livelihood of men is to be obtained from it. Again, Kama being the occupation of public women, they should prefer it to the other two. And these are exceptions to the general rule.'
—Kama Sutra *1.2.14[14]*[1]

What is the *Kama Sutra*? Is it a compendium of acrobatic sex positions—including one in which the man must stand on his head in the shirsha asana (a yogic headstand) to make love? Is it a guide to orgiastic excesses and delight, in which a man may satisfy three women at the same time? Is it a book for the courtesan? Is it a book of same-sex love? Is it a catalogue of aphrodisiacs which can keep men and women in a state of extended inebriated pleasure? Is it a how-to book which teaches men the means to enhance the size of their sexual organ and acquire immense prowess and energy?

The *Kama Sutra* is all of this and much more.

The *Kama Sutra* was compiled in the 4th century CE by the sage Vatsyayana, who is himself believed to have remained celibate all his life. It was brought to light in modern times by the British explorer Sir Richard F. Burton and translated by F. F. Arbuthnot from Sanskrit to English. First published by the Kama Shastra Society in 1883, its circulation was restricted

1. Sinha, Indra. *The Love Teachings of the Kama Sutra*, Bookwise: New Delhi, 2004-2005.

to a limited audience—publishing under the aegis of a private society was the only way to avoid censorship. It took more than eighty years, until 1962, for the *Kama Sutra* to be published in the Western world, so powerful were the vestiges of Victorian prudery in the English-speaking world.

There has always been a robust tradition of erotic writing in Indian literature—particularly in the genres of the Sanskrit kavya (poetry) favoured by court poets; Bhakti poetry and Sangam literature. In pre-modern India, there were several outstanding writers who composed poems, plays, novels, philosophical texts and works on the practice and theory of love. The wealth of this literature demonstrates that the erotic played an important role in the lives and the consciousness of people, and that the pleasure principle was of great significance in pre-modern India. Poems and plays freely chronicled love affairs, sexual adventures, faithfulness and infidelity. Both male and female beauty were celebrated—men were described as having 'great arms' like 'plantain trees', torsos 'like the face of an ox' and eyebrows 'like a strong bow'. Women, meanwhile, possessed faces 'like the full moon' and were 'long-eyed', 'tiny-waisted' and 'broad-hipped'. An instance of the centrality of the pleasure principle can be found in the *Gathasaptasati*, compiled by the Satavahana king Hala around the 2nd century BCE, which is perhaps the oldest extant anthology of poetry that has come down to us. Focusing on themes of love and the erotic, the anthology is quite extraordinary in its frank treatment of sexual desire and relationships.

In this context, the *Kama Sutra* may be described as a

distillation of the kama-related wisdom of India's enlightened pre-modern sages. One of the first sages to reflect on kama was Shvetaketu, the son of Uddalaka, who recorded a summary of Nandi's words in the 8th century BCE. Nandi, Shiva's sacred bull and his doorkeeper, is credited with having transmitted the very first treatise on lovemaking to mankind. According to tradition, Nandi overheard the sacred utterances of the god Shiva and his wife Parvati while they were making love. He then conveyed to mankind what had transpired between the divine couple within the divine bedchamber, and his description of this divine coupling formed the basis of the kama shastras.

Shvetaketu's scholarship was extensive, and a number of learned and holy men were deeply influenced and inspired by his work between the 3rd and the 1st centuries BCE. Babhravya, Charayana, Ghotakamukha, Gonardiya, Gonikaputra, Suvarnanabha and Dattaka are only a few of many such scholars and sages. It is said that Vatsyayana drew upon all their ideas to compile the *Kama Sutra*.

One of the source texts in the Indian kama shastra tradition—works dealing with sexual pleasure in the Indian literary tradition—the *Kama Sutra* is, to my mind, the mother of all erotic manuals across continents and cultures. Within India itself, it inspired a number of erotic texts, such as the *Koka Shastra* and the *Ananga Ranga*, both of which were written in the medieval period and are significant in their own right. If the *Artha Shastra* is the defining text which covers the principles of politics and governance, the kama shastras instruct the *nagarika*, or sophisticated townsman, on matters of pleasure.

In Indian culture and philosophy, the ideal life is guided by a judicious balance of the four *purusharthas*, or goals of life: *dharma* or righteousness, *artha* or the creation of wealth, *kama* or the fulfillment of desires and, the final goal, *moksha* or spiritual liberation. The first three must be well balanced for any individual to eventually achieve the fourth, *moksha*. Therefore, Vatsyayana emphasizes, although the *Kama Sutra* focuses on just one goal, this does not mean that life should be spent only in the pursuit of pleasure. At the end of the book, the author suggests that the *Kama Sutra* should be read and understood in the correct context, and not seen merely as a hedonistic instruction manual written solely for pleasure seekers.

In their translation of the *Kama Sutra*, Wendy Doniger and Sudhir Kakar describe the *Kama Sutra* thus: 'It is not the sort of book to read in bed while drinking heavily, let alone holding the book with one hand in order to keep the other free (...) The *Kama Sutra* is an ancient Indian textbook about sex—in the very broadest sense of the word. *Kama* means love, pleasure, sex, while *sutra* means a treatise, or a scientific work. It is about the whole eroticized world of pleasure, so it's about food and soft moonlight and good music and flowers strewn all over the bedroom. It is also about meeting people: how you meet someone you're going to marry, how you meet someone you're not going to marry, how you deal with a married woman or a married man, and so forth. It's about the whole web of interpersonal relationships, which has an erotic basis'.

In this small intimate book of images, appropriately named *The Little Book of Pleasure*, I am looking at four concepts through which I would like to unpack the colossus which is the *Kama Sutra*. In order to get a taste of the aesthetics of the erotic and the exploration of desire from which stems kama (pleasure), I am taking you, dear reader, through the love escapades of the *nayaka* and the *nayika*, and through *maithuna* where the sexual act gives *ananda* or ultimate joy which is aided and abetted by the *ganika* or the courtesan.

The *Kama Sutra* is one of the world's most widely illustrated texts. Almost all illustrated versions available today, however, are products of a refined brush, and therefore, while exquisite, also predictable. This selection is a deliberate deviation towards a raw, almost primitive representation. The images in this little book will surprise you with their naïve quality, which is unique to the Sirohi School of miniature painting from Rajasthan.

There are also a few photographs here, from the collection of an early twentieth-century Rajasthani aristocrat, that share the naïve quality of the paintings. These photographs were taken by a man who was, like Vatsyayan himself, an artist, a voyeur, an aesthete. The models who posed for him were probably from his staff. Did they pose for him willingly or because they dare not refuse? Did they do it for money, for pleasure, for the sheer novelty, or for all of these reasons? Who can tell? Desire takes many forms. I like to think that whatever the nature of the transaction, it gave everyone pleasure—the performers, the artist, the voyeur.

May this little book give you pleasure, too.

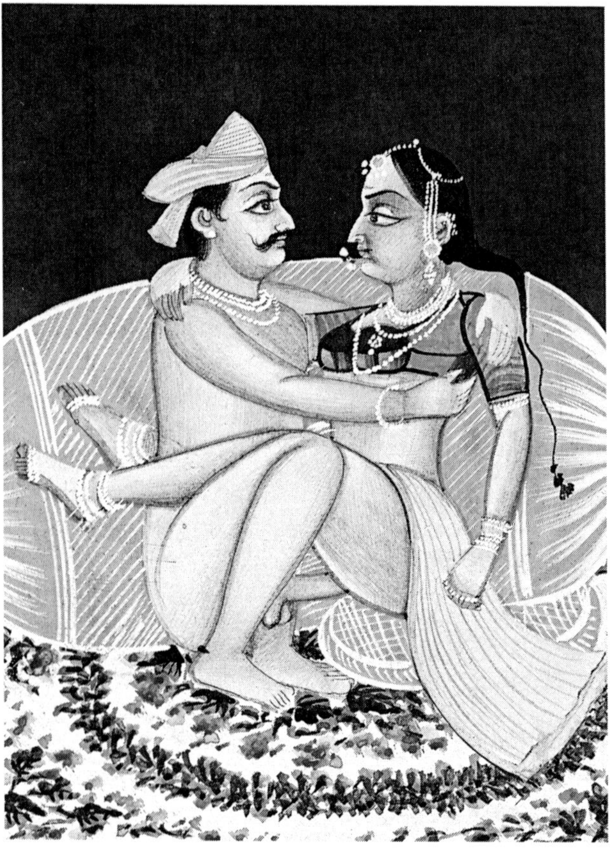

Zone of comfort, Nathdwara School, 19th century, natural pigments with gold flange on paper.

Nayaka/Nayika

Comparing the *Kama Sutra* with Sanskrit drama, Wendy Doniger and Sudhir Kakar point out that it has a hero (*nayaka*) and a heroine (*nayika*), as well as stock characters: the sidekick, the supporting player and the jester. The text of the *Kama Sutra* also reads like a play in that the plot unfolds through a series of dialogues and soliloquies. In addition, it follows the seven-act format of most classical Indian dramatic works. Act One has the hero establishing his bachelor pad; in Act Two, he perfects his techniques. Act Three finds him seducing a virgin and getting married. In Act Four, he lives with a wife or wives, but tires of them, so he seduces other men's wives (Act Five) and then moves on to courtesans (Act Six). Finally, when age and physical decay interfere with his fun, he turns to magic spells and aphrodisiacs (Act Seven).

The *Kama Sutra* classifies the *nayaka* and the *nayika* into three categories, depending on the size of their genitals; within each category, men and women can further be divided into three more categories depending on their sexual temperament. Finally, their degree of skill in love-making makes them fall into a further three categories, creating an incredible array of possibilities for better or less satisfying sexual intercourse.

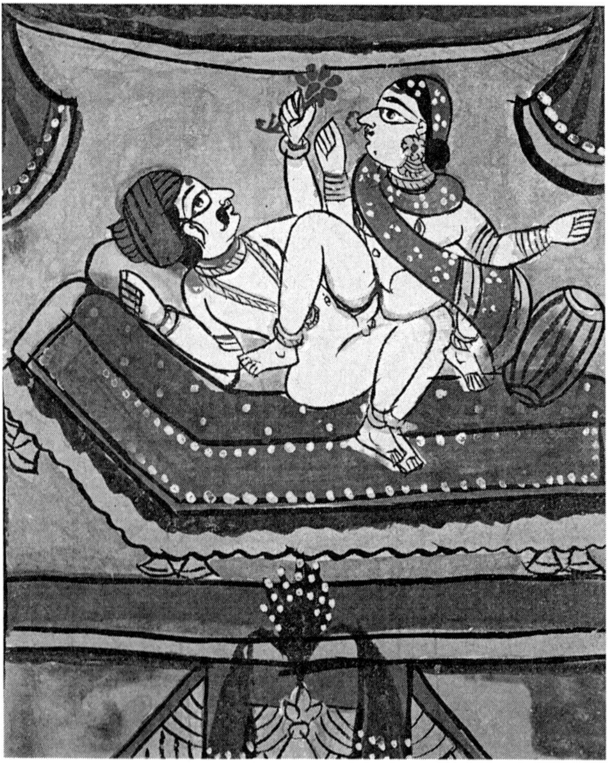

Top: *Say it with flowers*, Sirohi School, early 19th century, natural pigments on paper.

Opp: *A casual encounter,* Sirohi School, early 19th century, natural pigments on paper.

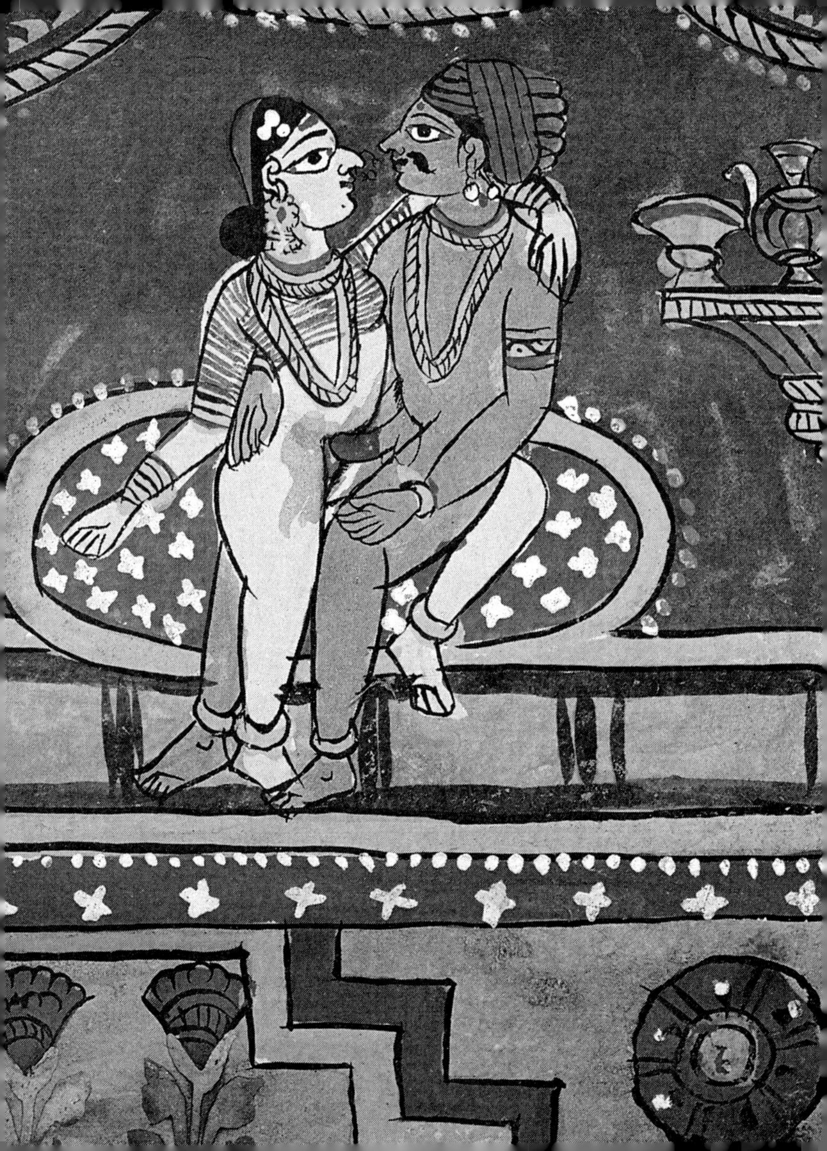

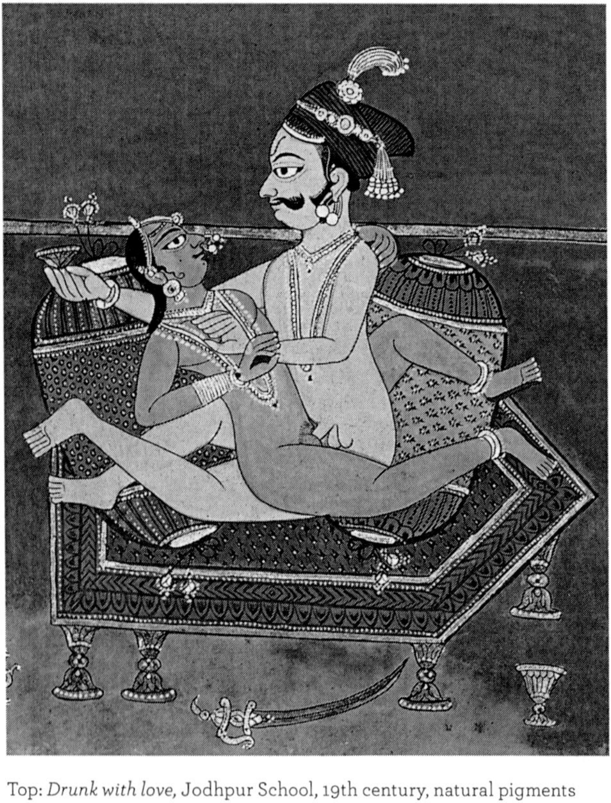

Top: *Drunk with love,* Jodhpur School, 19th century, natural pigments with gold flange on paper.

Opp: *Playing with the pillow,* Jodhpur School, 19th century, natural pigments with gold flange on paper.

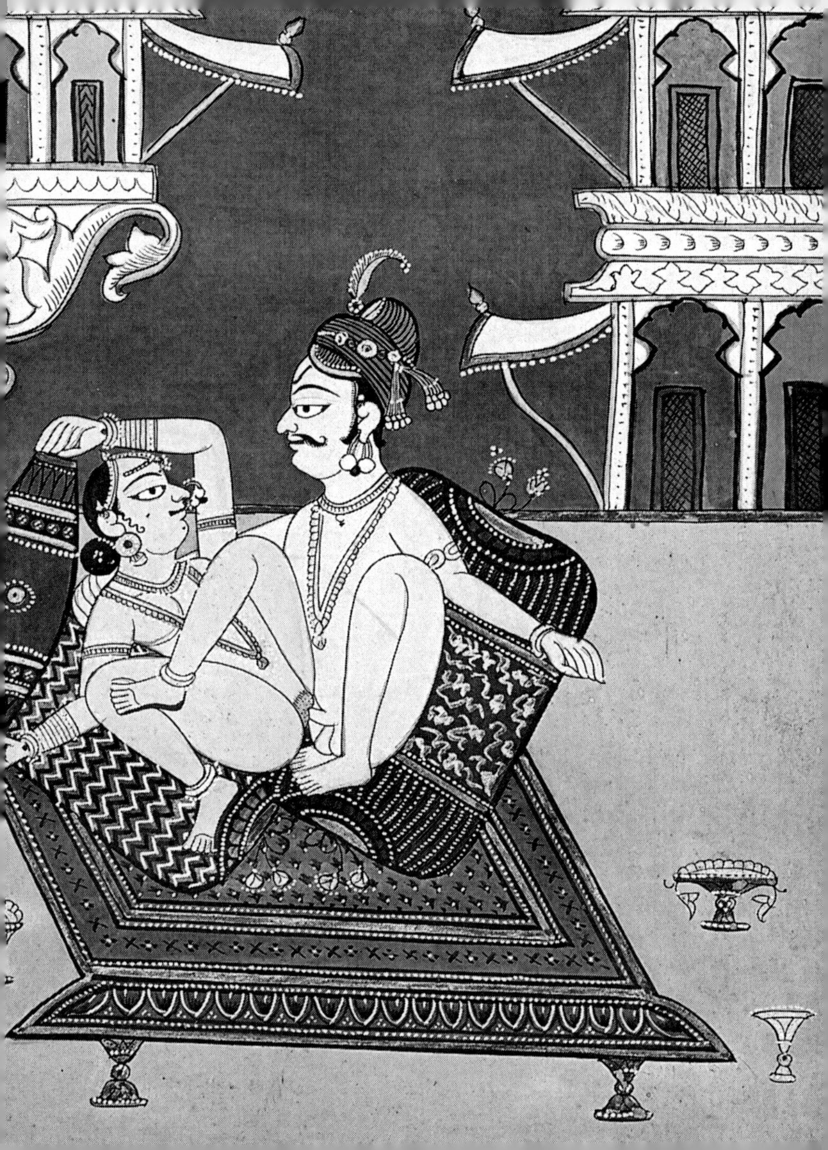

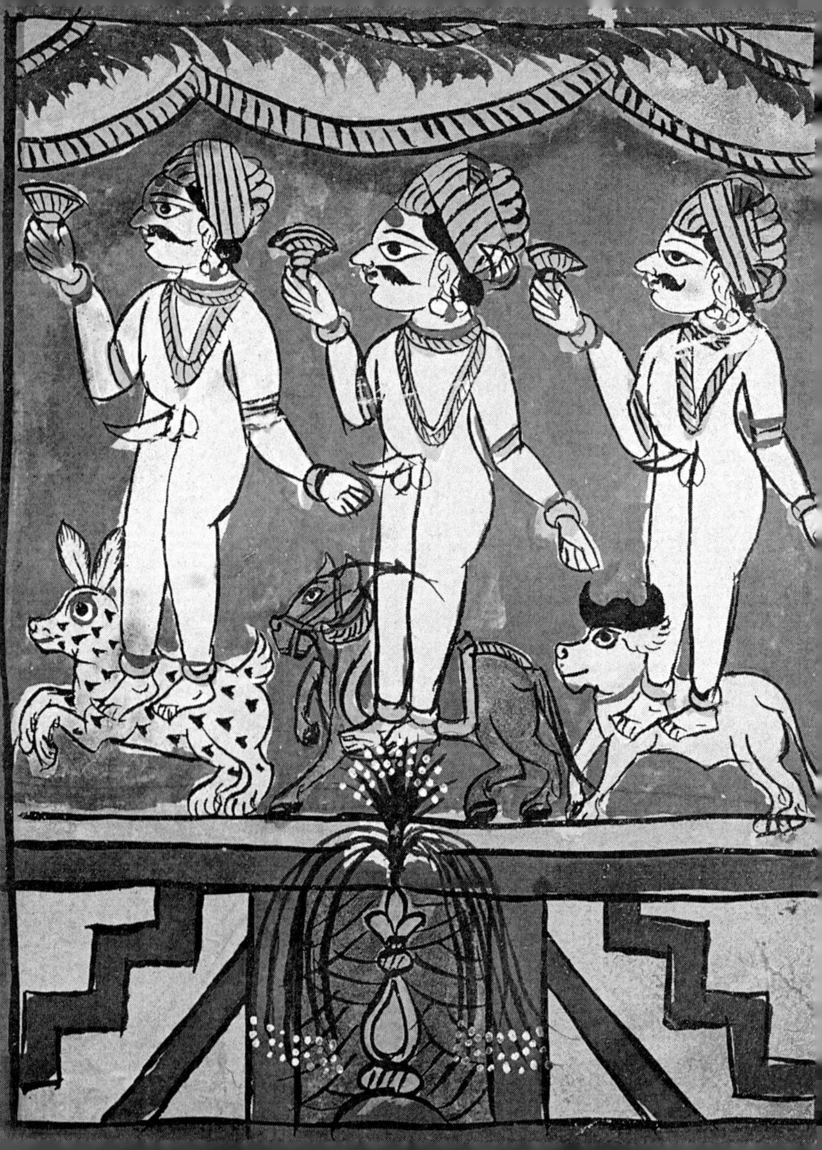

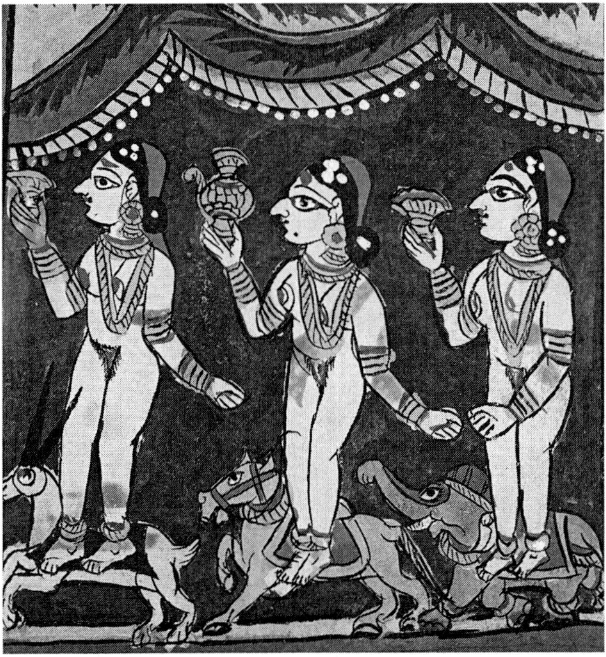

Top: *The dog, the mare, and the elephant,* Sirohi School, early 19th century, natural pigments on paper.

Vatsyayana classifies women as does, mares, or elephants depending on the depth of their yoni (vagina), and matched with their male equivalent, it leads to more or less 'compatible' couplings.

Opp: *The hare, the horse and the bull,* Sirohi School, early 19th century, natural pigments on paper.

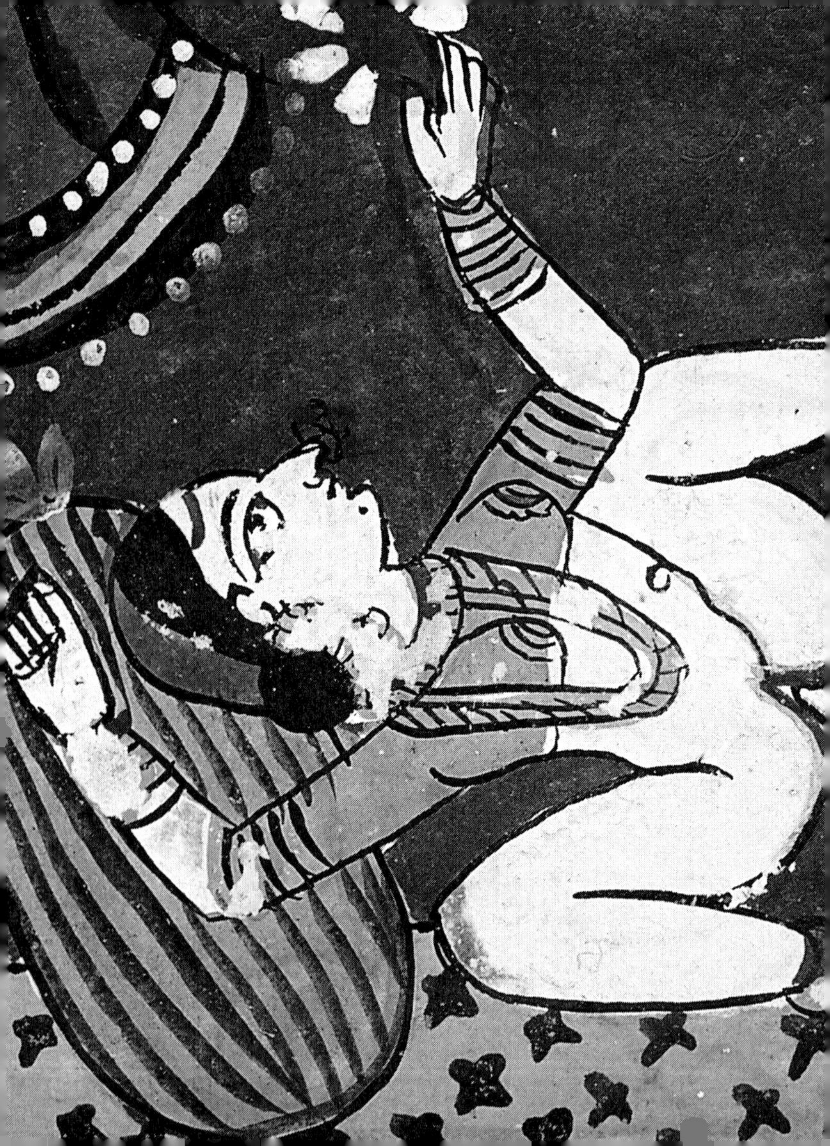

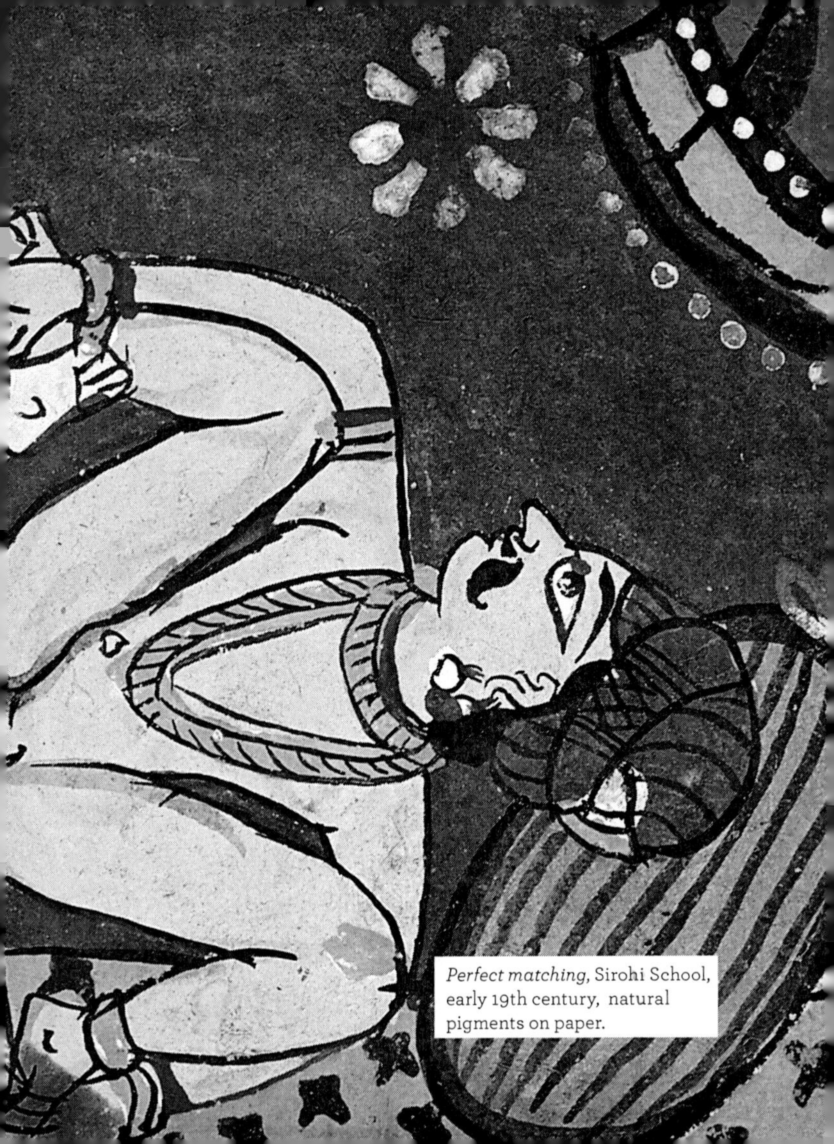

Perfect matching, Sirohi School, early 19th century, natural pigments on paper.

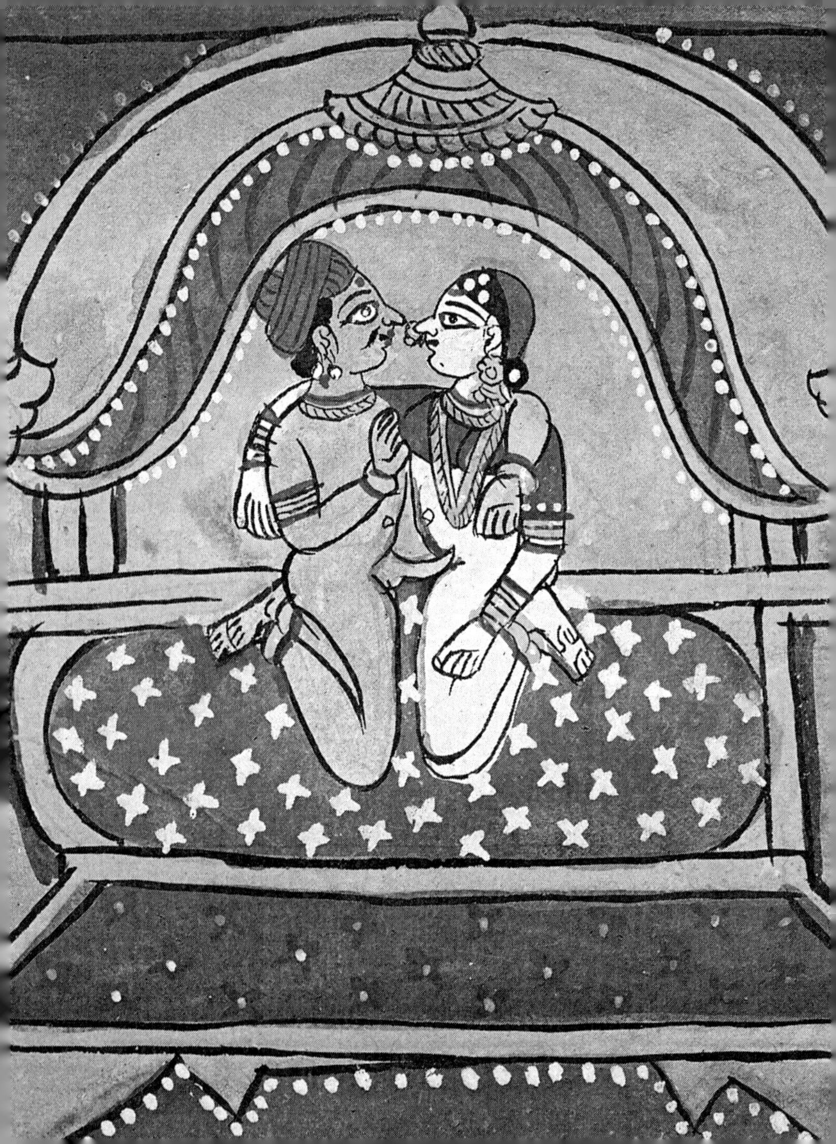

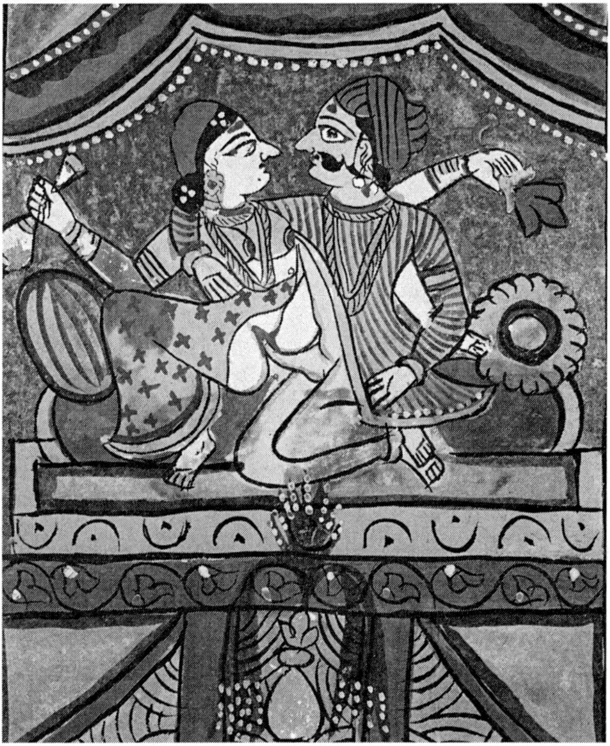

Top: *Taken by surprise,* Sirohi School, early 19th century, natural pigments on paper.

Opp: *Comfortable with each other,* Sirohi School, early 19th century, natural pigments on paper.

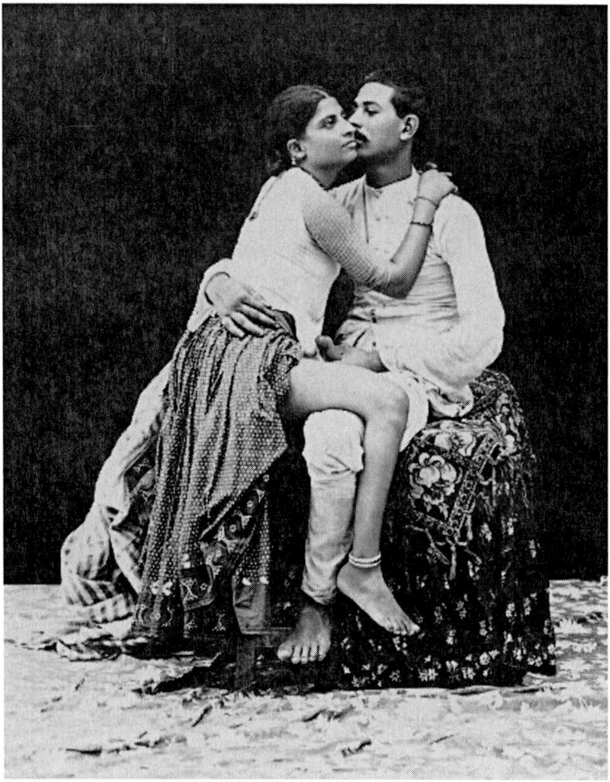

Discovering each other, photo album from the Royal House of Kutch, 1890-1900.

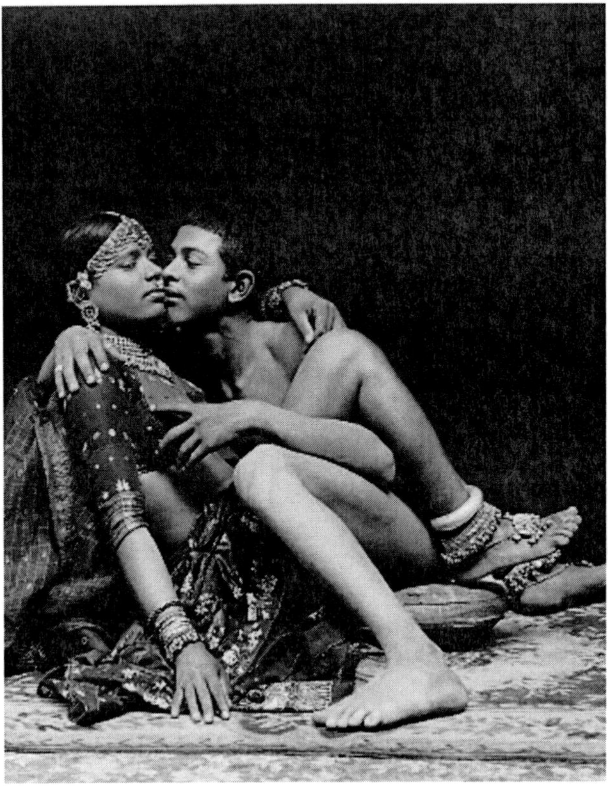

A recurring trope, photo album from the Royal House of Kutch, 1890-1900.

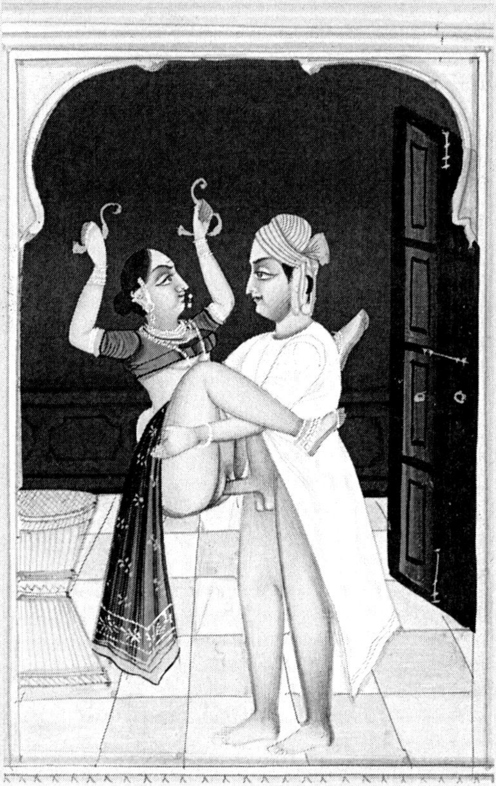

Hanging with joy, Nathdwara School,19th century, natural pigments with gold flange on paper.

The skill of a lover depends on how much he can prolong lovemaking because every woman like men who can pleasure them for hours, says Vatsyayana in the Kama Sutra.

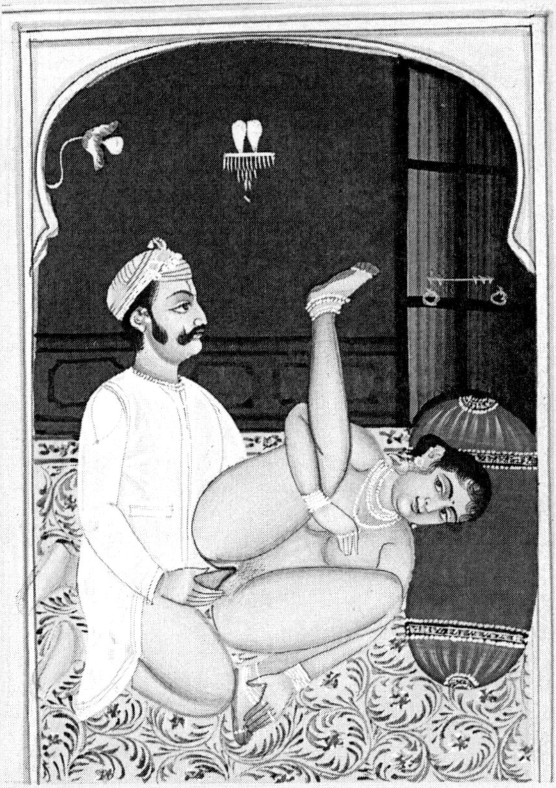

The supple and the skilled, Nathdwara school, 19th century, natural pigments with gold flange on paper.

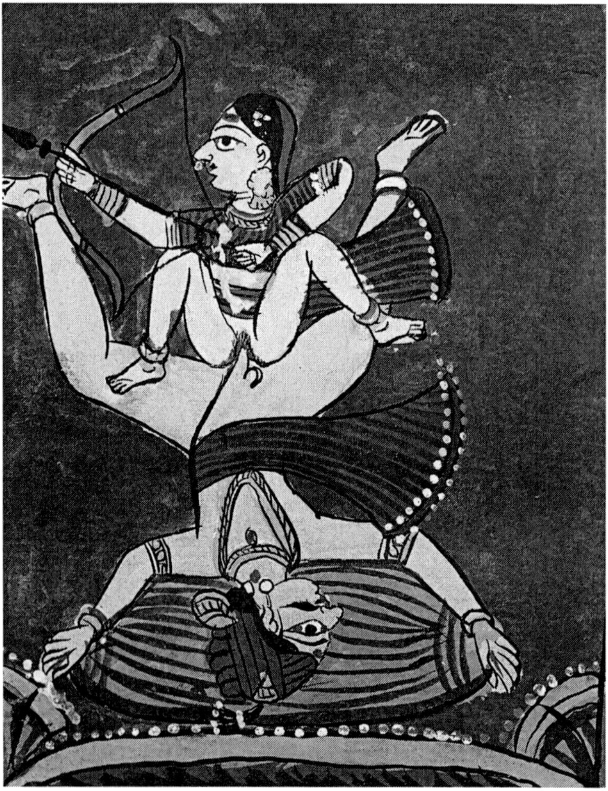

The skilled archeress, Sirohi School, early 19th century, natural pigments on paper.

Maithuna

Within the Hindu tradition, erotic play and sexual union is embedded in the divine, the spiritual and the temporal. The lovemaking of the gods is frequently mentioned—the most significant example being the graphic descriptions of the sexual congress of Shiva and Parvati which, when overheard by Shiva's doorkeeper Nandi, became the bases for the writing of the *Kama Sutra*. In *grihastha ashram*, the second or householder phase of an individual's life, sex is an important part of procreation as well as pleasure.

Acquiring knowledge in the domain of sex was very much a part of every young urban sophisticate's coming of age. Studying the *Kama Sutra*, or the discipline of kama (pleasure), was an essential part of a refined education in Ancient India. The urban sophisticate citizen or *nagarika* was not only well versed in the art of business and commerce but also in the aesthetics of love-making, seduction and *maithuna* or sexual congress.

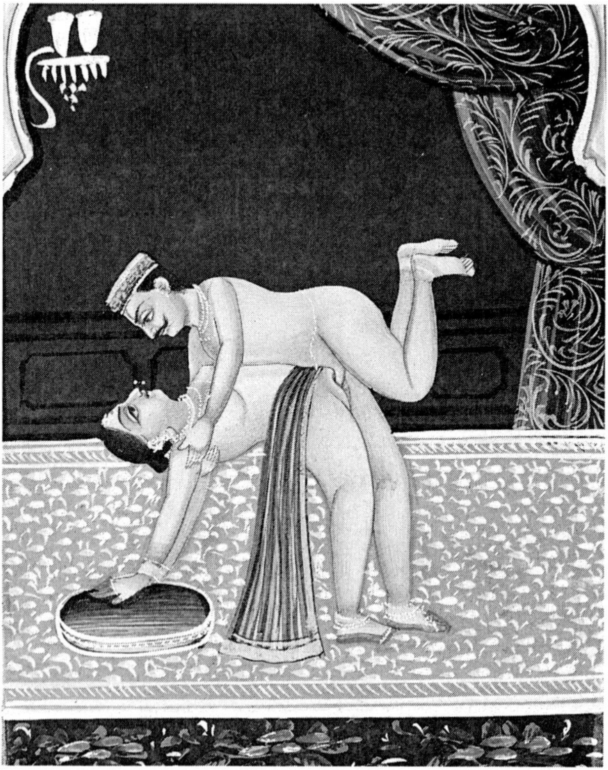

In cosy harmony, Nathdwara School, 19th century, natural pigments with gold flange on paper.

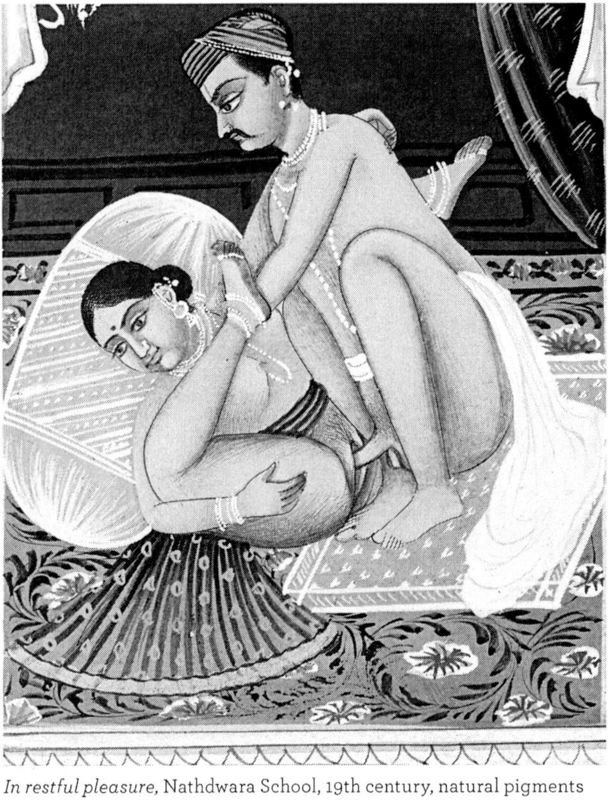

In restful pleasure, Nathdwara School, 19th century, natural pigments with gold flange on paper.

The series of paintings make use of the common trope of the curtain being lifted up so as to reveal the erotic scene happening behind. It gives a sense of subtle voyeurism to increase the pleasure of the viewer.

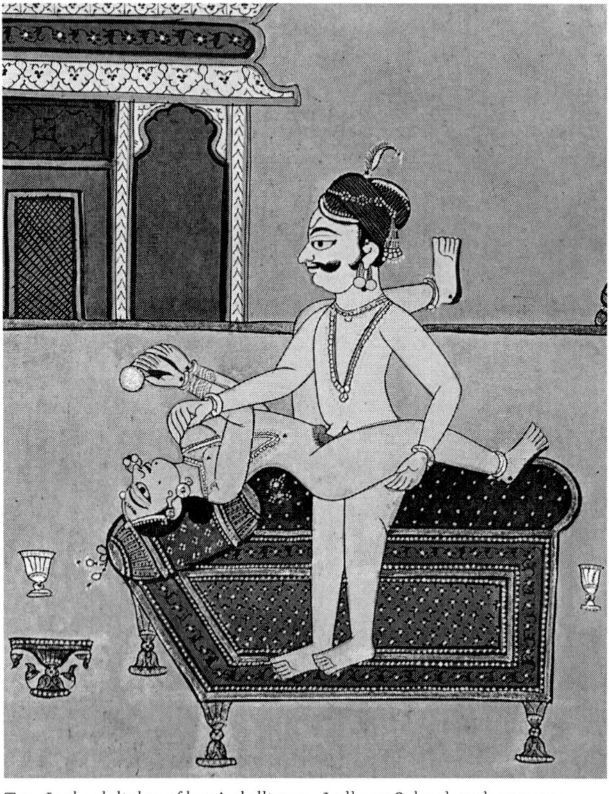

Top: *In the delights of love's dalliance,* Jodhpur School, 19th century, natural pigments with gold flange on paper.

Opp: *In the velvet darkness of the night,* Jaipur School, c. 1780, natural pigments with gold flange on paper.

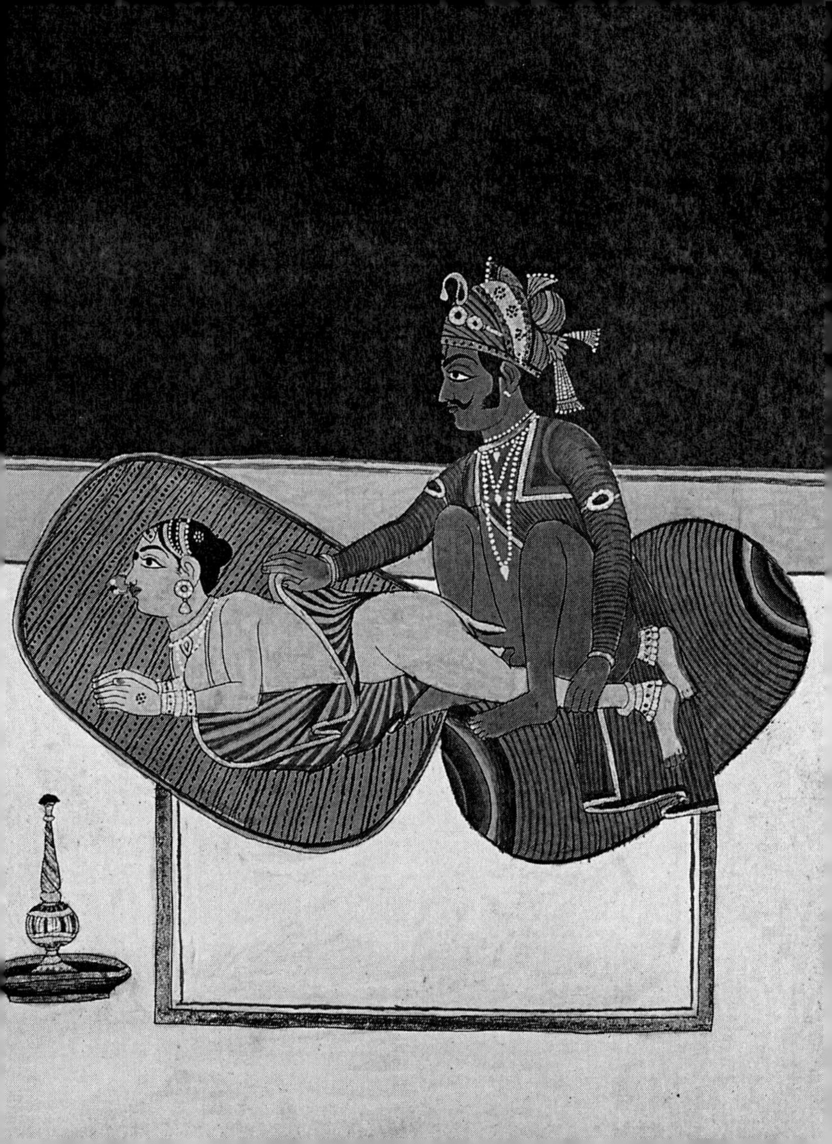

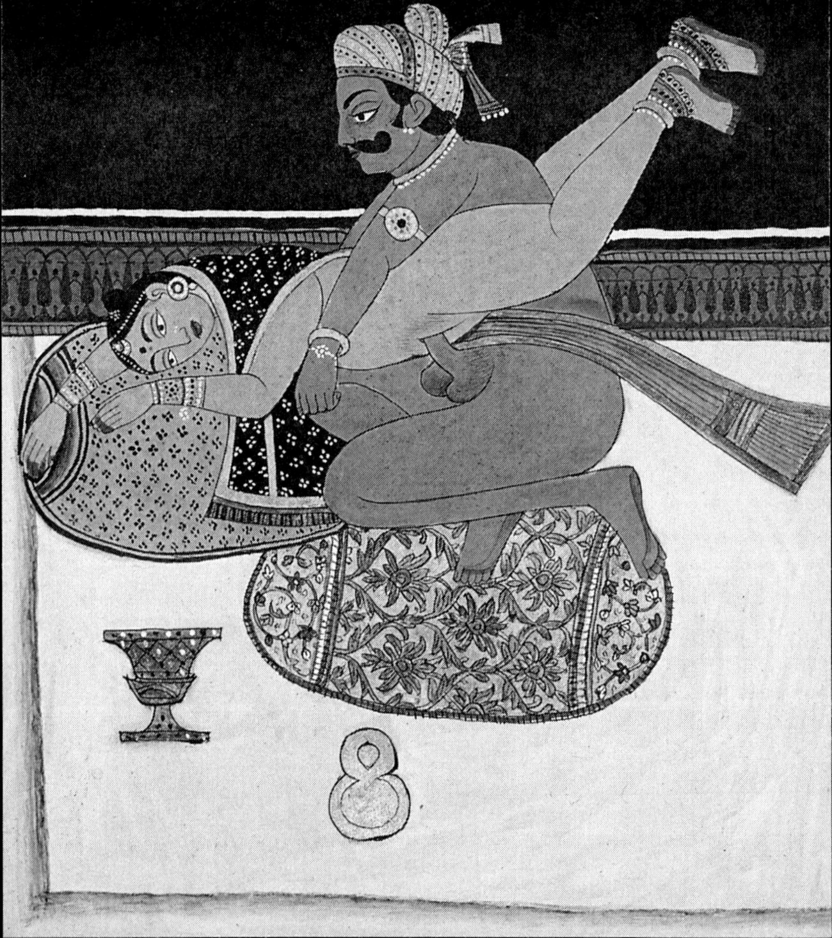
8

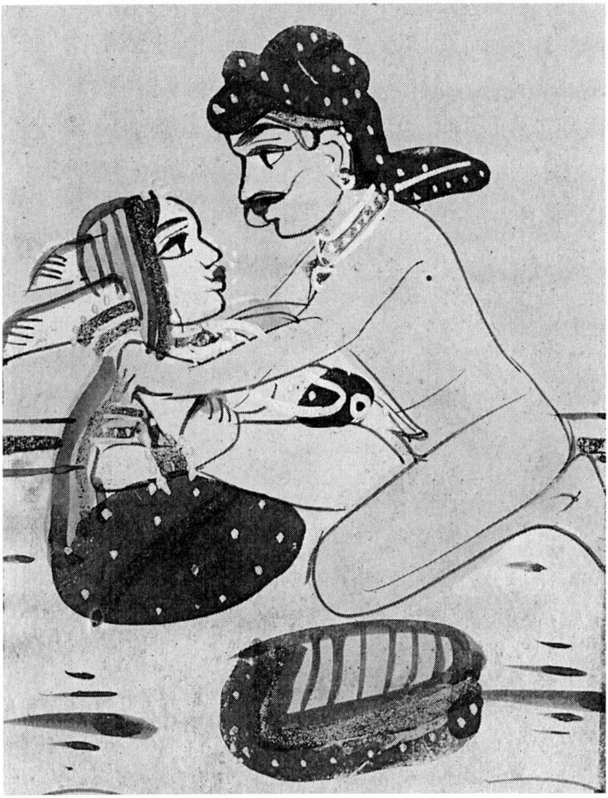

Top: *Man in control,* Jaipur School, c.1880, natural pigments on paper.

Opp: *The powerful patron,* Jaipur School, c. 1780, natural pigments with gold flange on paper.

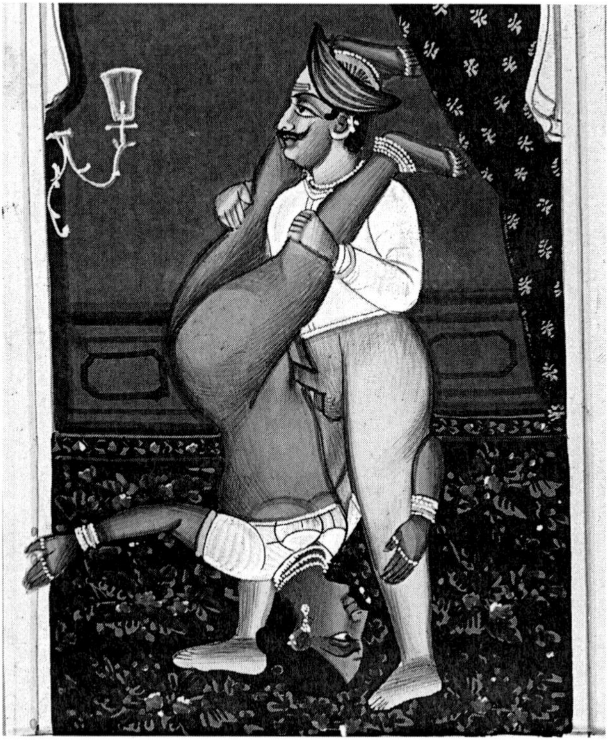

Acrobatic dalliance, Nathdwara School, 19th century, natural pigments with gold flange on paper.

Opp: *Tenderness,* Nathdwara School, 19th century, natural pigments with gold flange on paper.

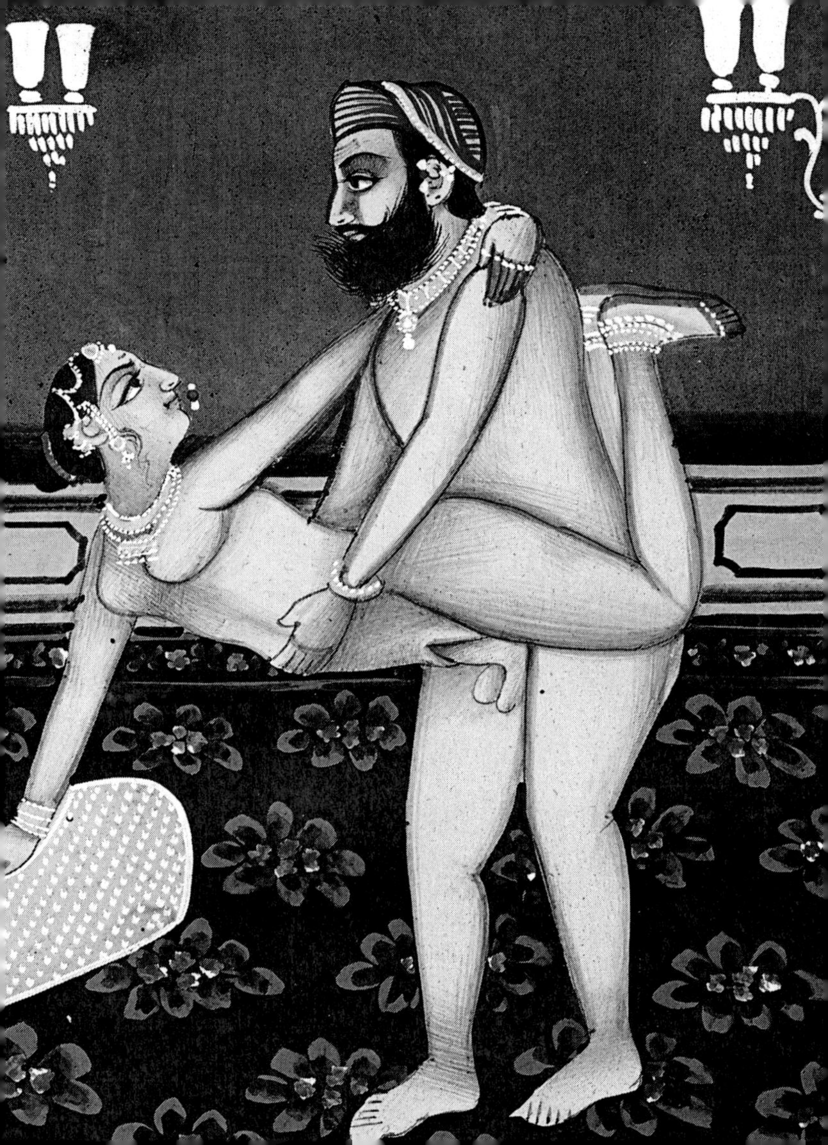

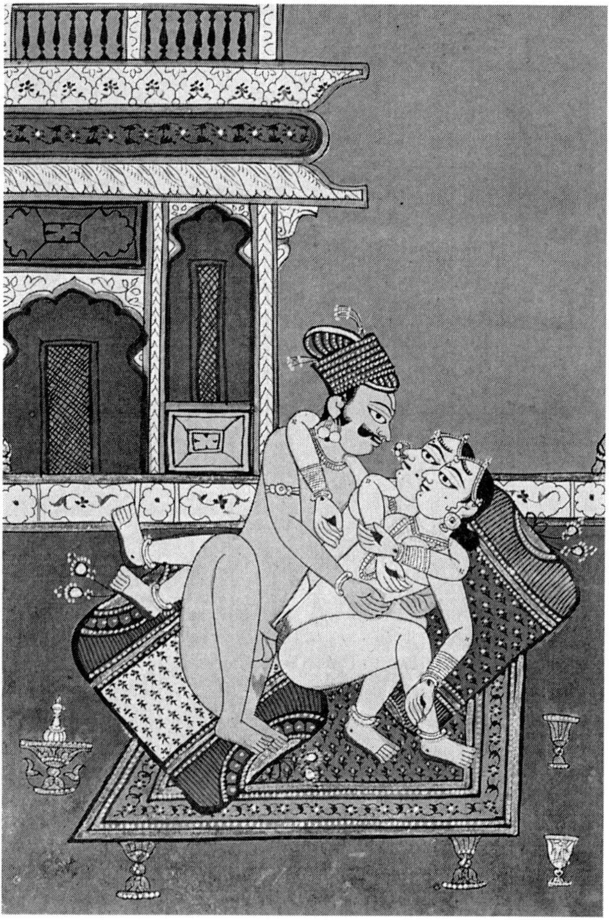

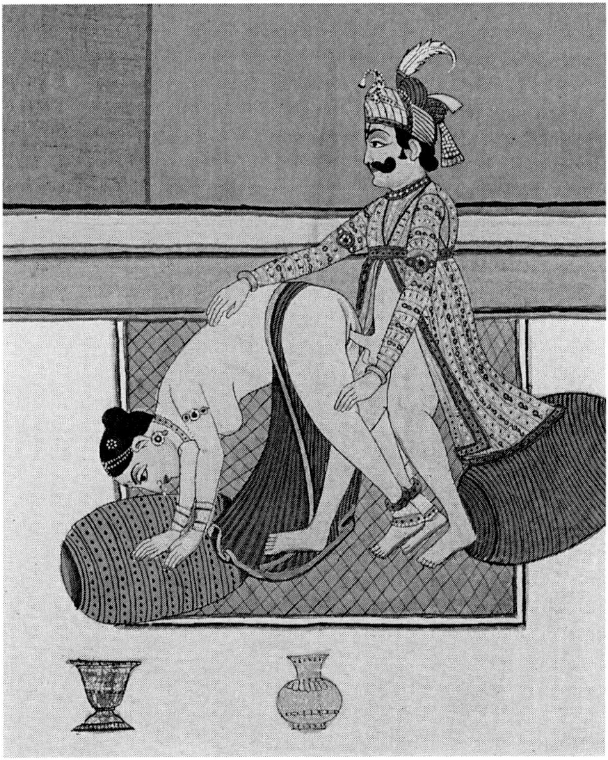

In a new environment, Jaipur School, c. 1780, natural pigments with gold flange on paper.

Opp: *Double the pleasure,* Jodhpur School, 19th century, natural pigments with gold flange on paper.

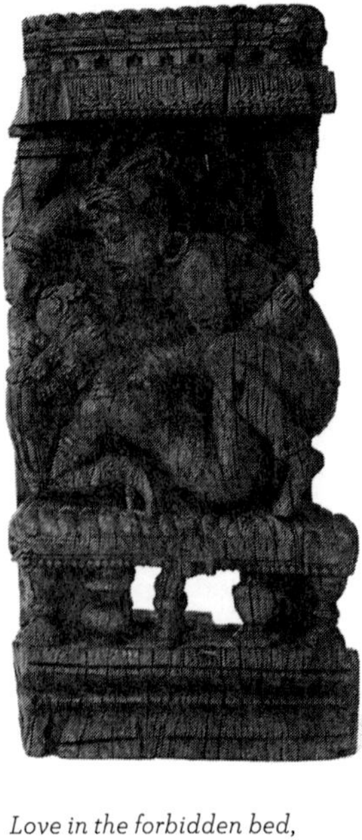

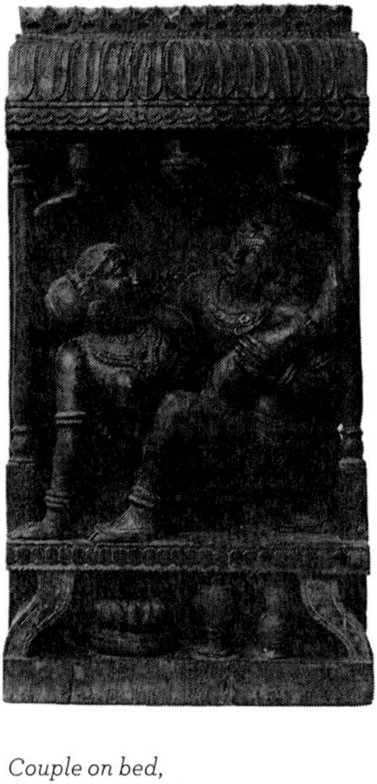

Love in the forbidden bed,
Tamil Nadu, 19th century,
wood carving

Couple on bed,
Tamil Nadu, 19th century,
wood carving

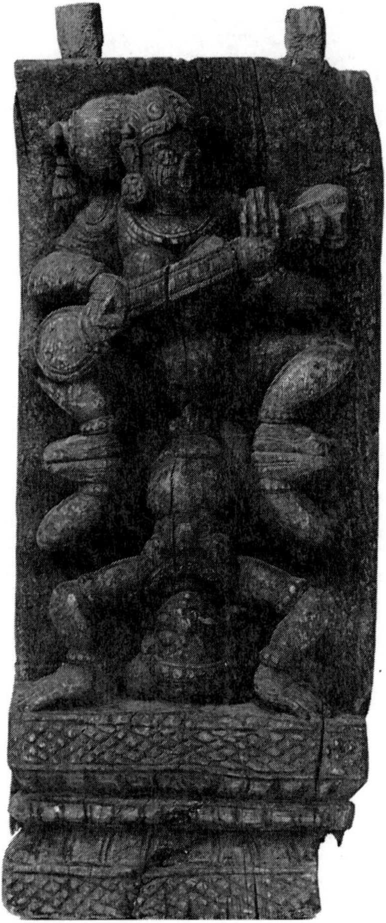

On a headstand,
Tamil Nadu, 19th century,
wood carving

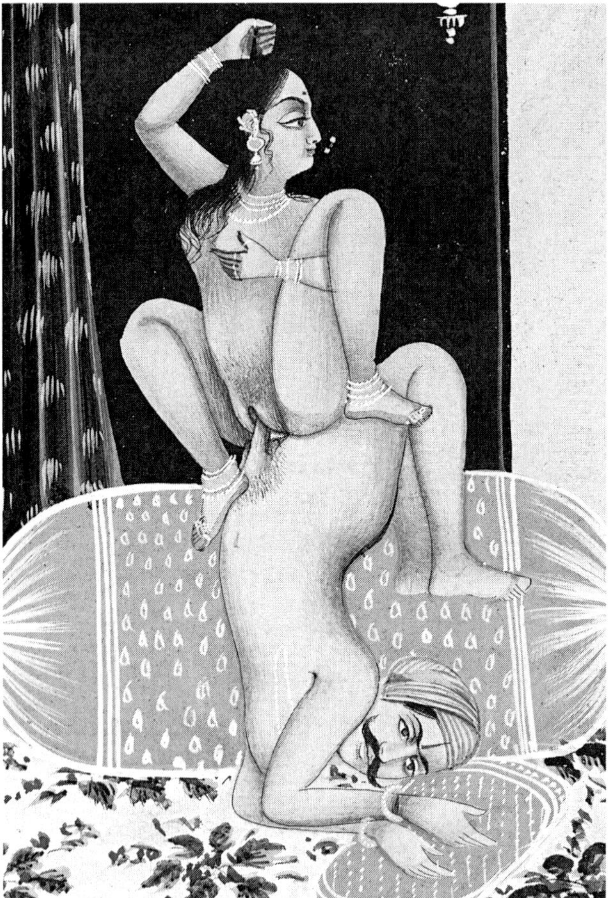

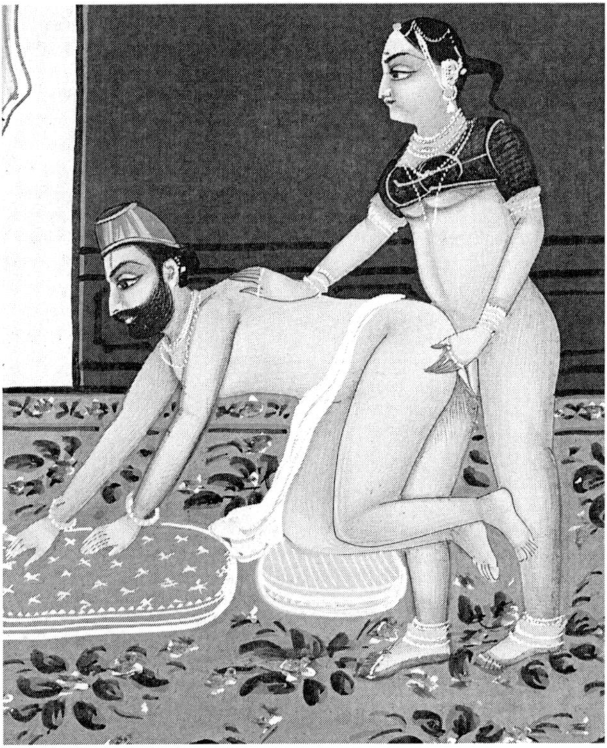

Taking the man's role, Nathdwara School, 19th century, natural pigments with gold flange on paper.

Opp: *Absorbed in pleasure,* Nathdwara School, 19th century, natural pigments with gold flange on paper.

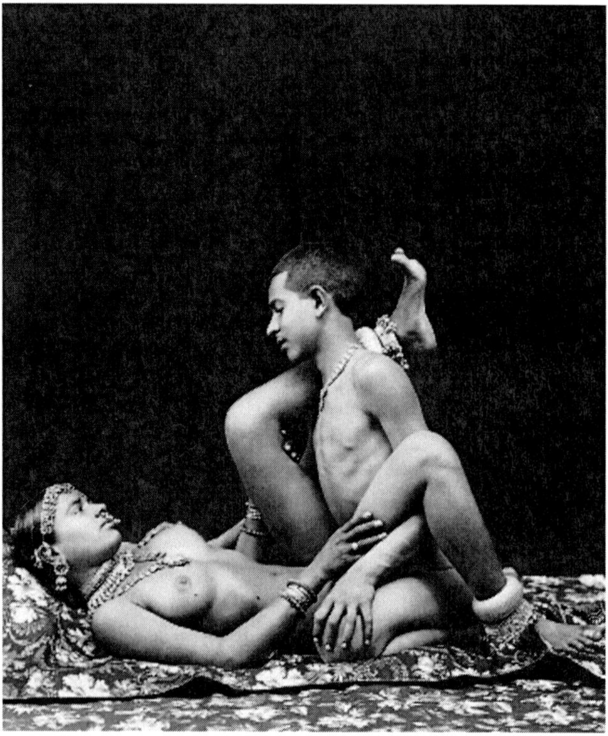

The first flush of physical joy, photo album from the Royal House of Kutch, 1890-1900.

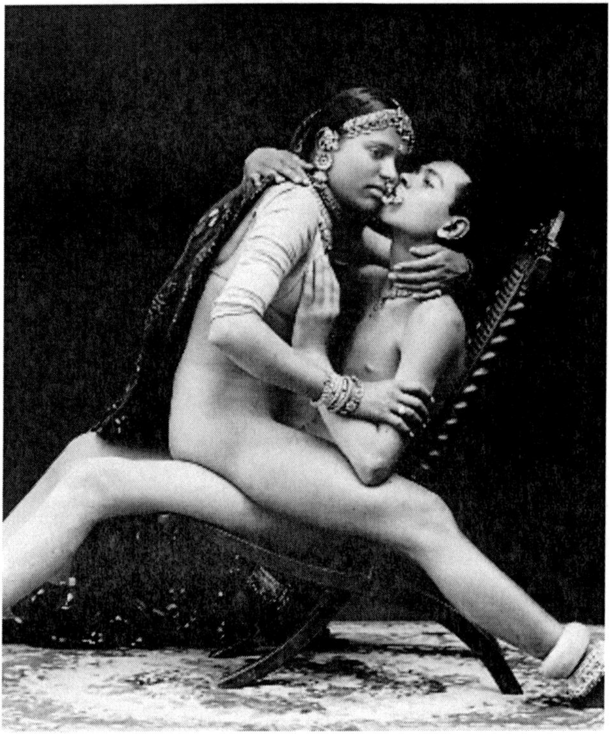

Youthful encounters, photo album from the Royal House of Kutch, 1890-1900.

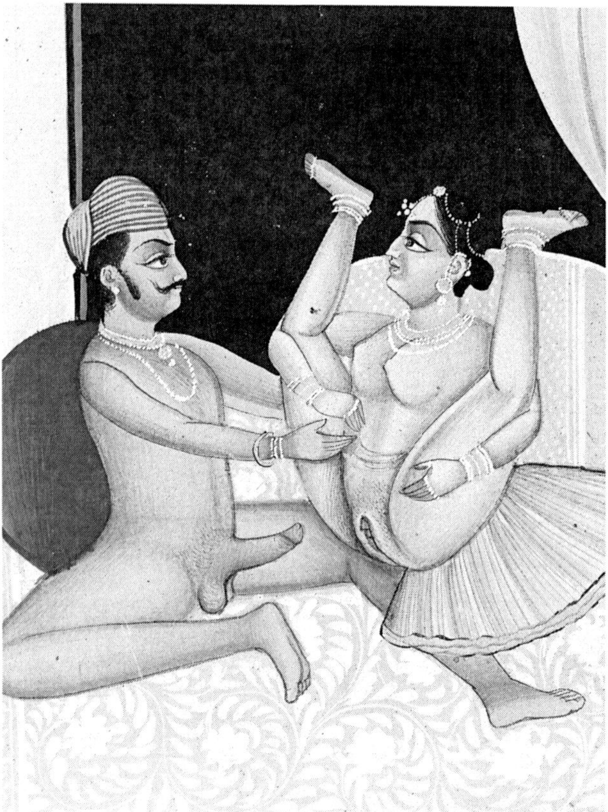

Ganika at her skillful best, Nathdwara School, 19th century, natural pigments with gold flange on paper.

Ganika

As the one who has mastered the art of Kama, the role of the *ganika* or courtesan becomes very important; it is the courtesans who trained the young *nagarika* or urban sophisticate citizen in the art of love-making, seduction, and, finally, satisfying the passions of their beloveds and paramours.

The *Kama Sutra* provides an exhaustive list of accomplishments a courtesan was expected to have. Aside from music, dance, acting and singing, she was to be well versed in architecture, clay modelling, composing poetry, different languages and in philosophy. She also had to know how to perfectly arrange flowers, to make perfumes and cosmetics, perform conjuring tricks, create riddles and tongue twisters; she had to be skilled at embroidery, cooking and gardening. She even had to be able to teach parrots and mynahs to talk.

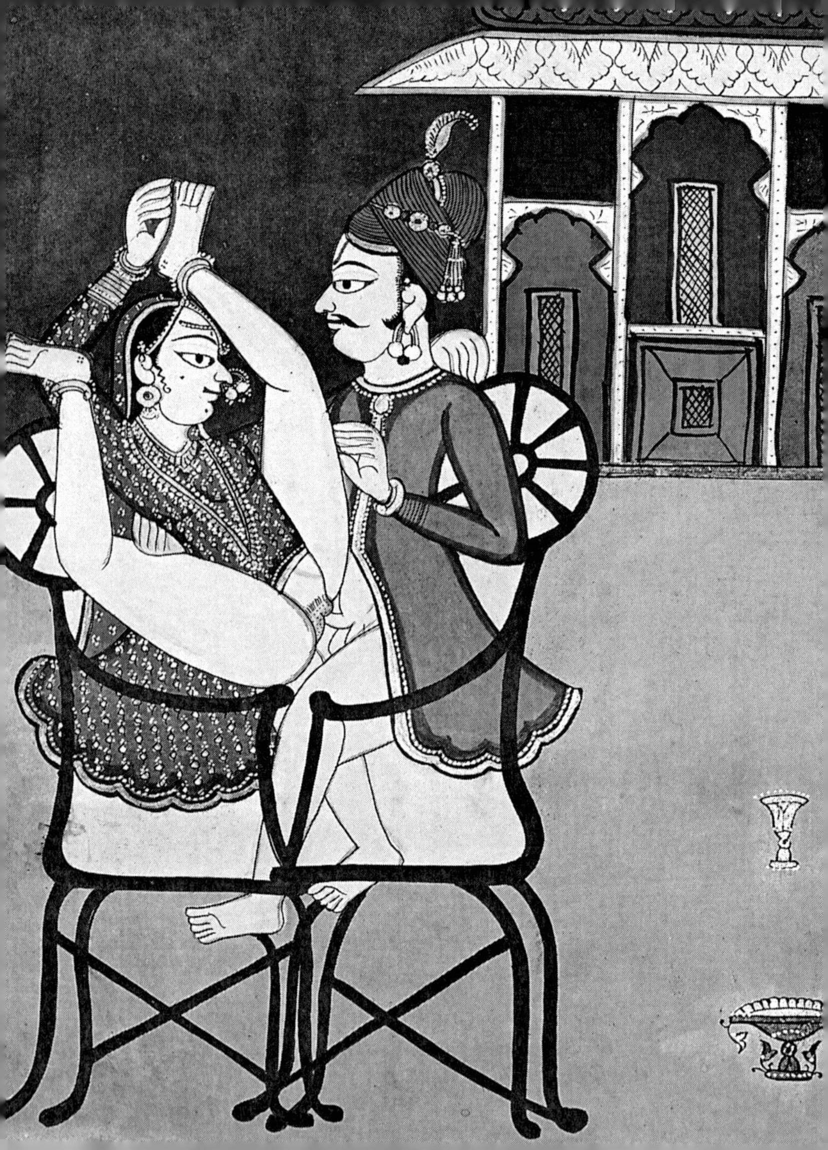

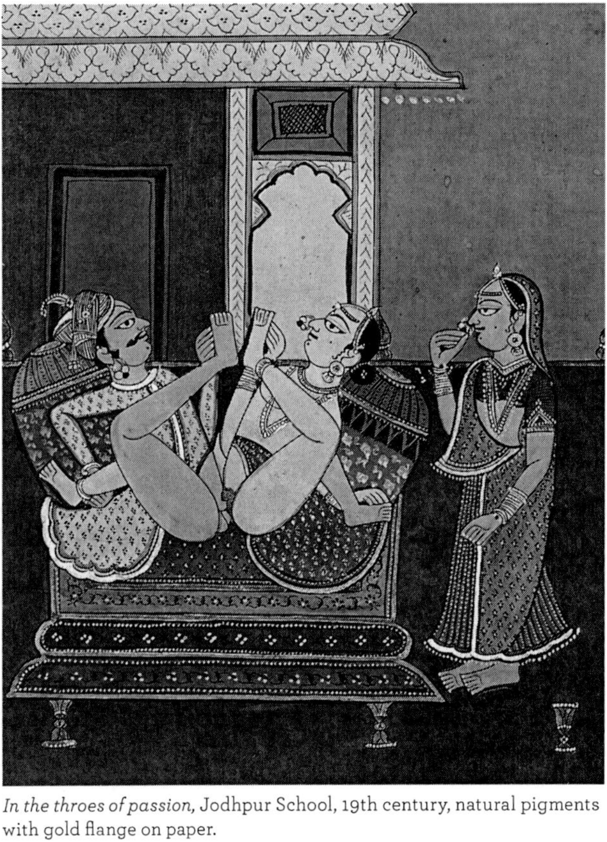

In the throes of passion, Jodhpur School, 19th century, natural pigments with gold flange on paper.

Opp: *Loveplay in a chair,* Jodhpur School, 19th century, natural pigments with gold flange on paper.

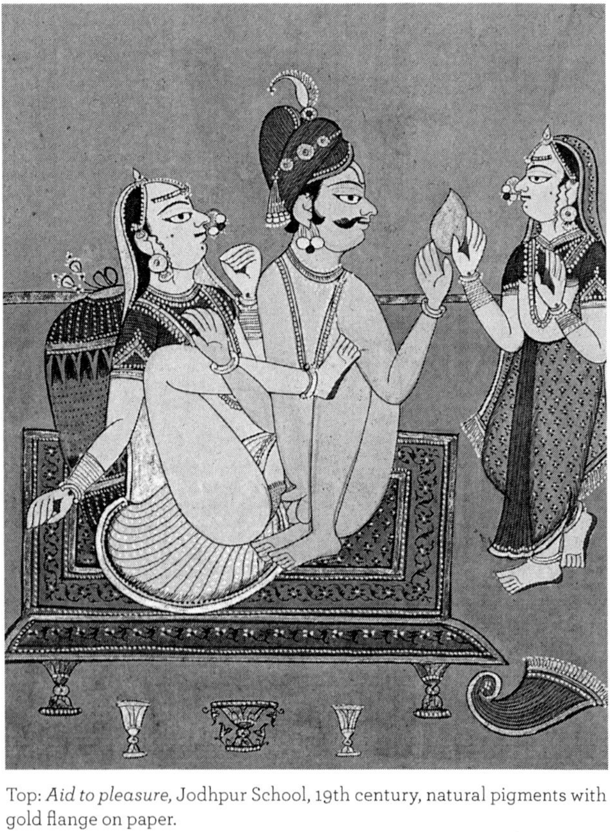

Top: *Aid to pleasure,* Jodhpur School, 19th century, natural pigments with gold flange on paper.

Opp: *The entanglements of love,* Jodhpur School, 19th century, natural pigments with gold flange on paper.

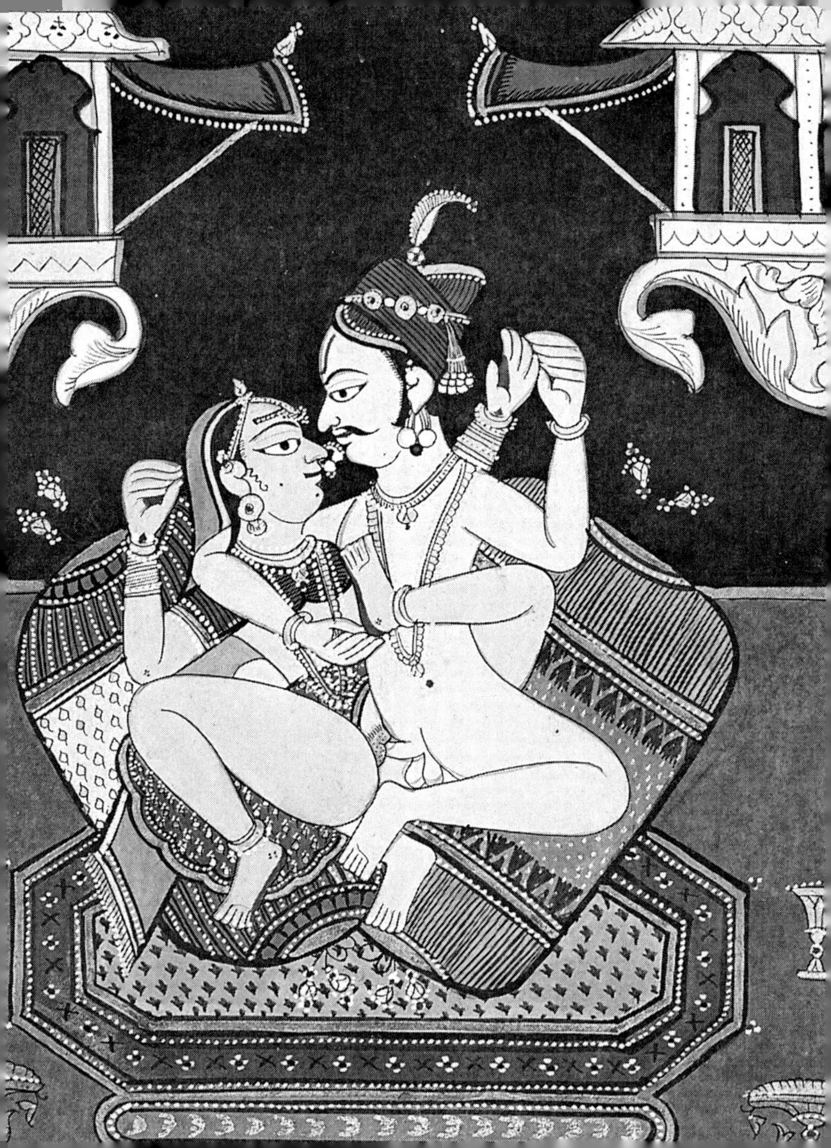

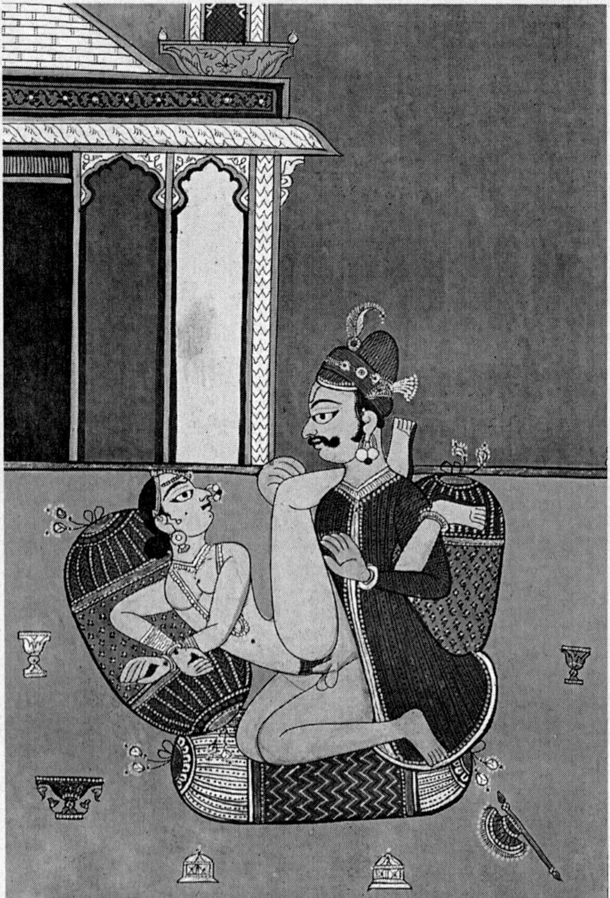

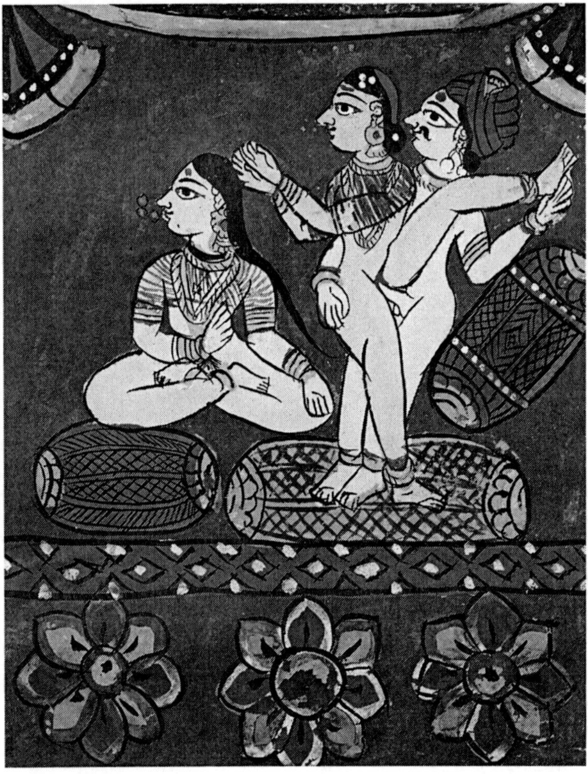

Top: *Distracted,* Sirohi School, early 19th century, natural pigments on paper.

Opp: *The supple damsel with her wealthy lover,* Jodhpur School, 19th century, natural pigments with gold flange on paper.

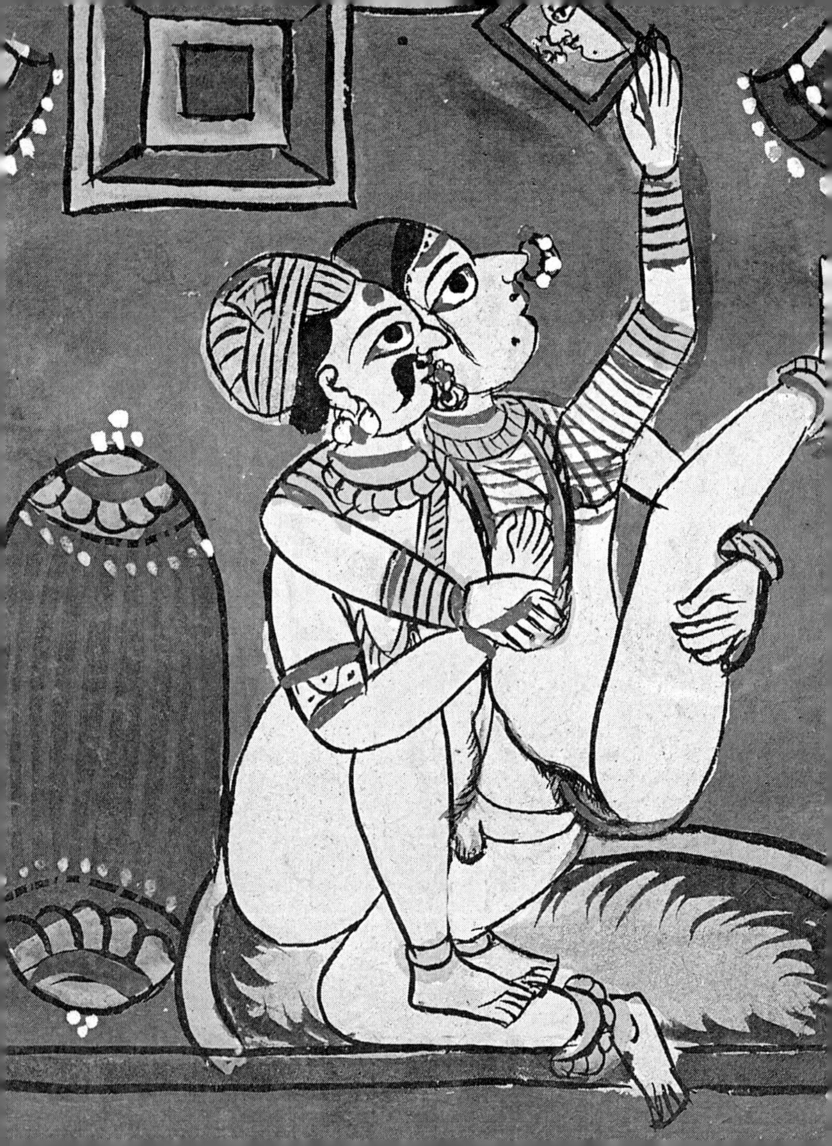

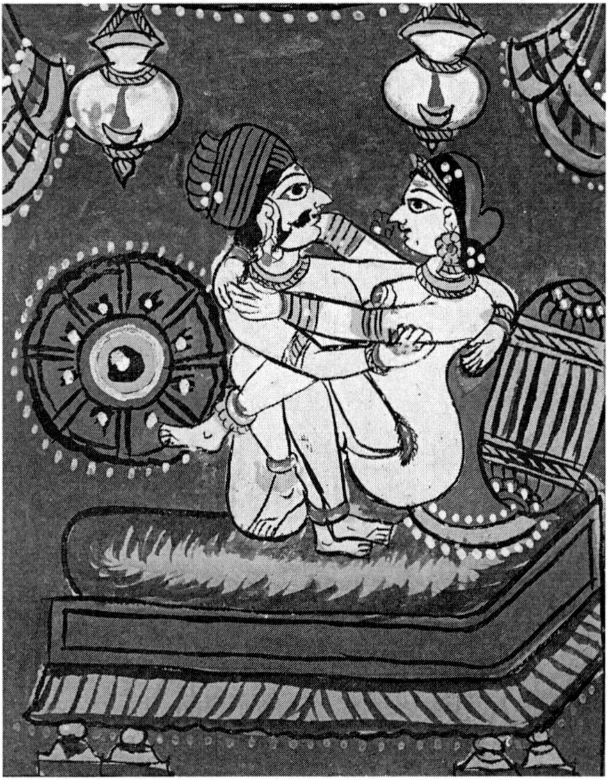

Top: *In close embrace,* Sirohi School, early 19th century, natural pigments on paper.

Opp: *Mirroring love,* Sirohi School, early 19th century, natural pigments on paper.

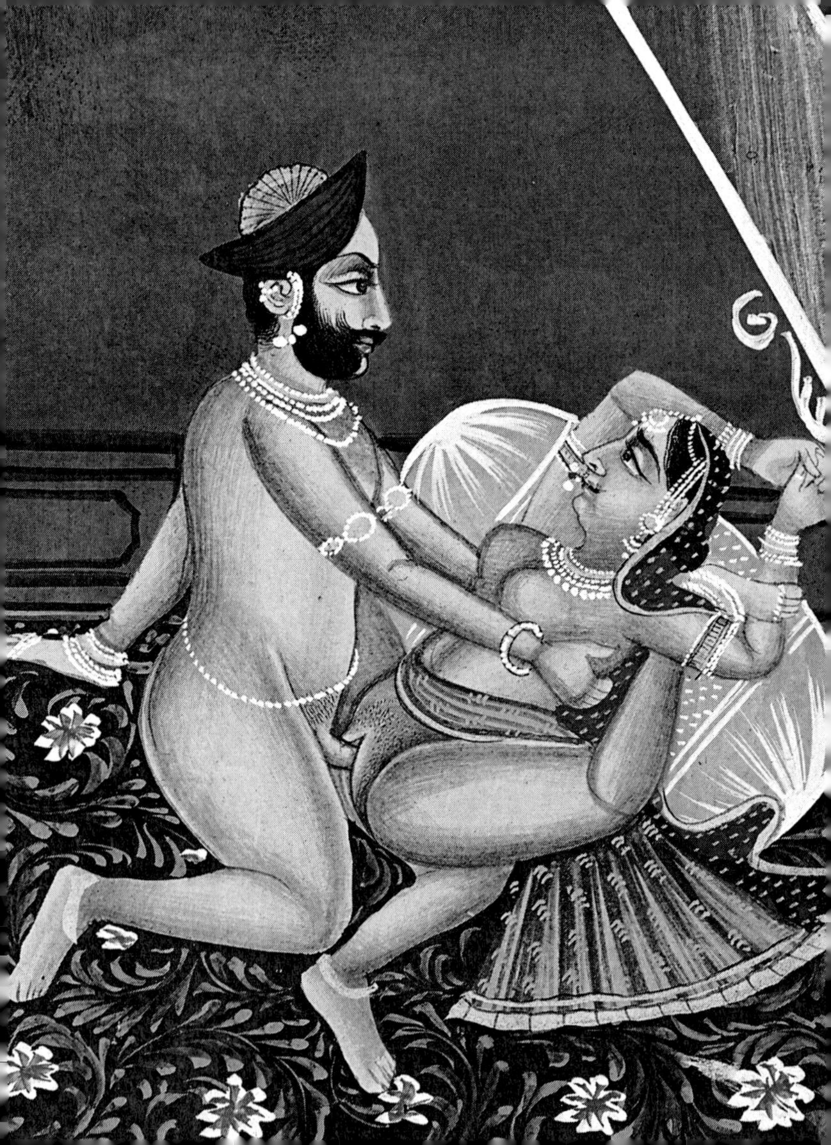

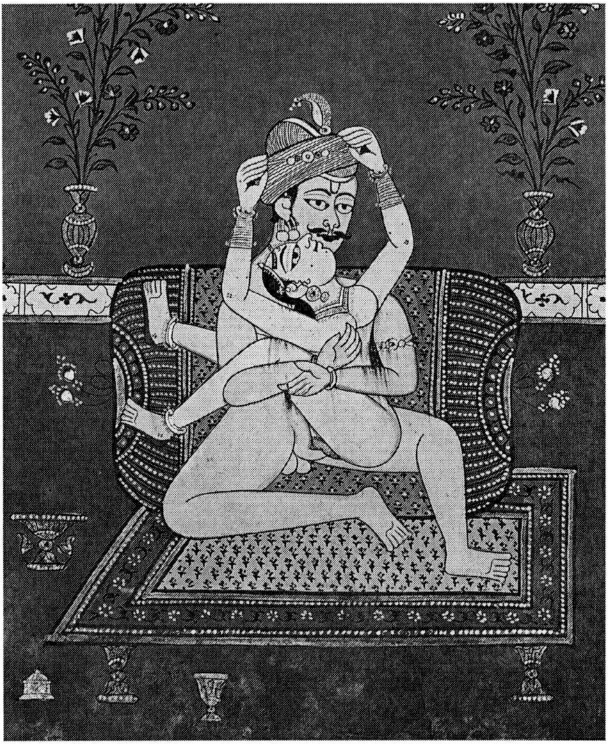

Top: *Adjusting the hat with love,* Jodhpur School, 19th century, natural pigments with gold flange on paper.

Opp: *The look of engagement,* Nathdwara school, 19th century, natural pigments with gold flange on paper.

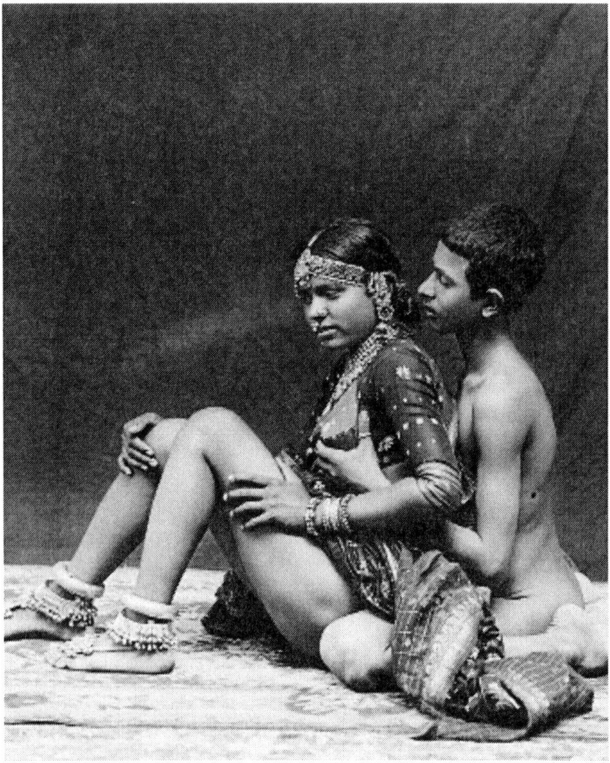

An emblem of desire, photo album from the Royal House of Kutch, 1890-1900.

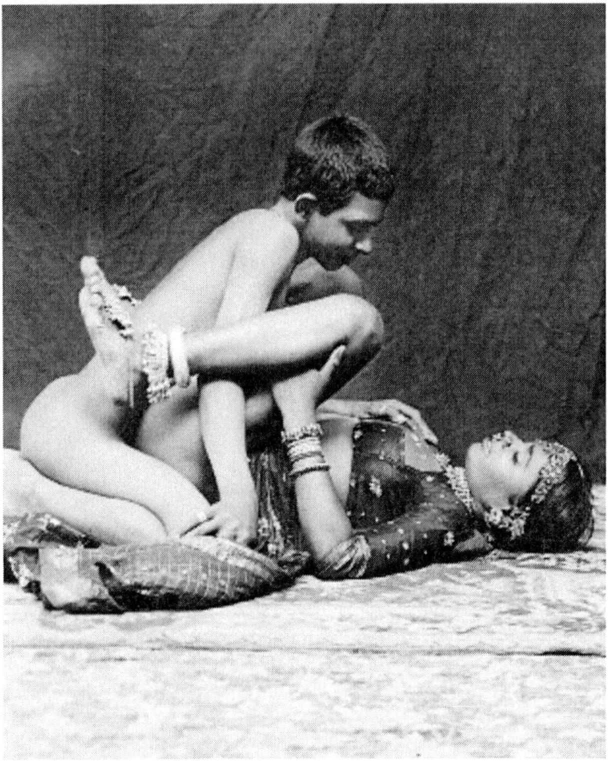

Staging sex, photo album from the Royal House of Kutch, 1890-1900.

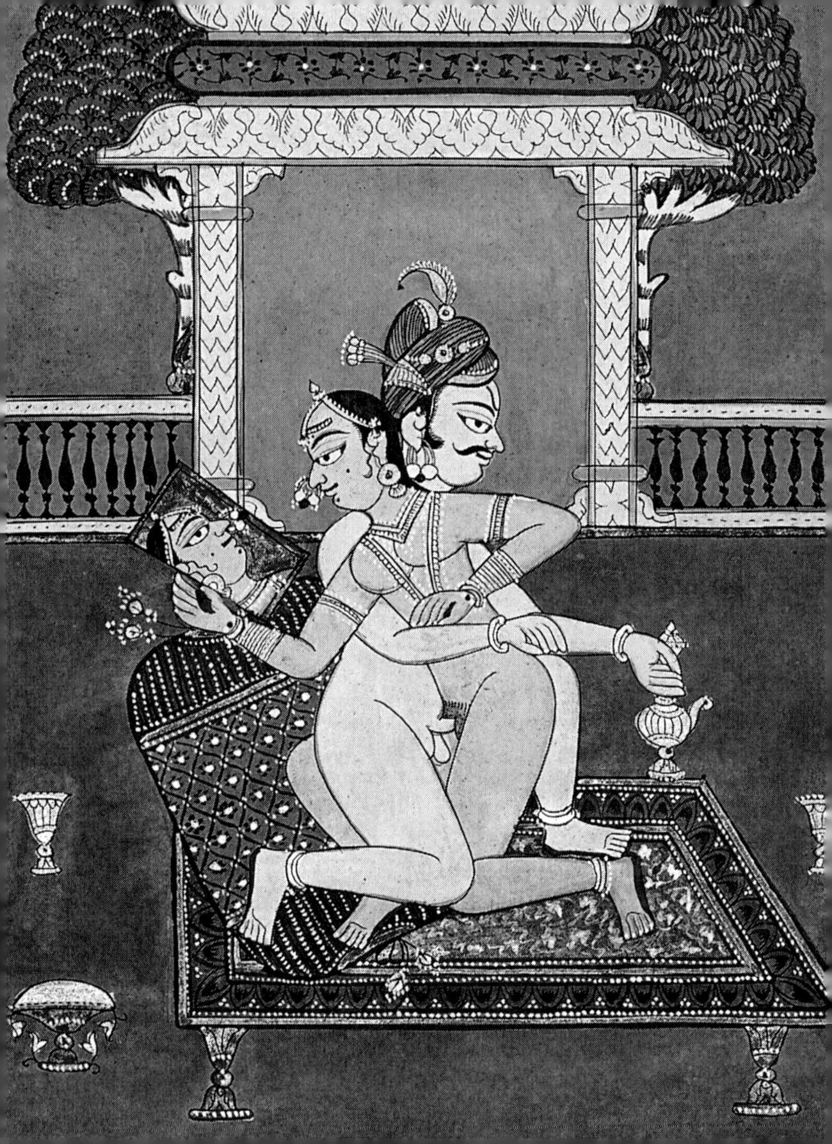

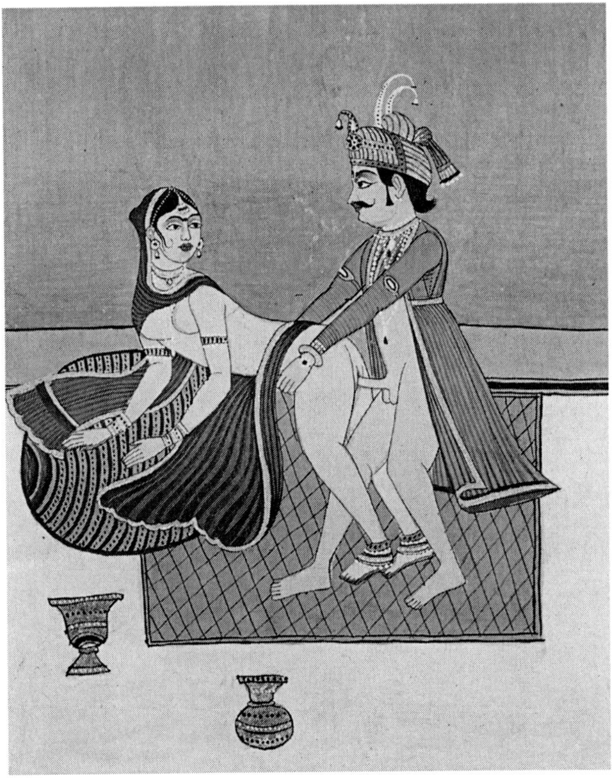

Top: *Unabashed in the act of love,* Jaipur School, c. 1780, natural pigments with gold flange on paper.

Opp: *The narcissist and her lover,* Jodhpur School, 19th century, natural pigments with gold flange on paper.

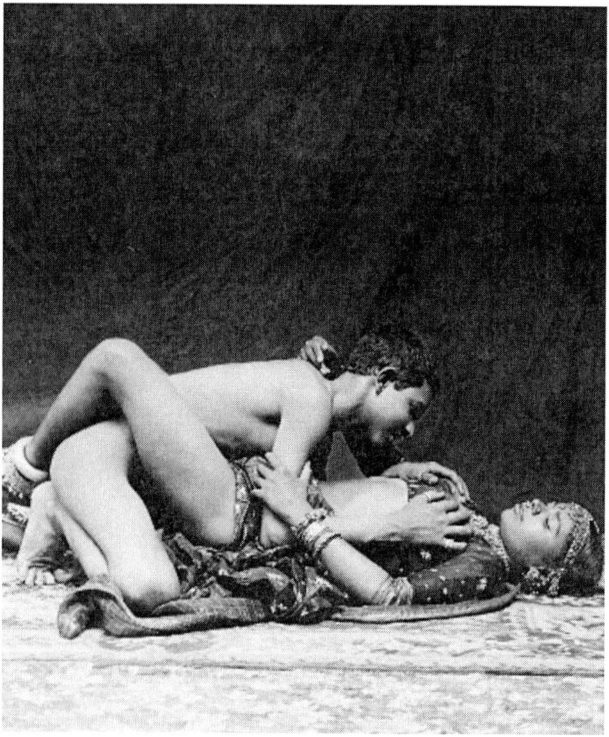

Between the sacred and the profane, photo album from the Royal House of Kutch, 1890-1900.

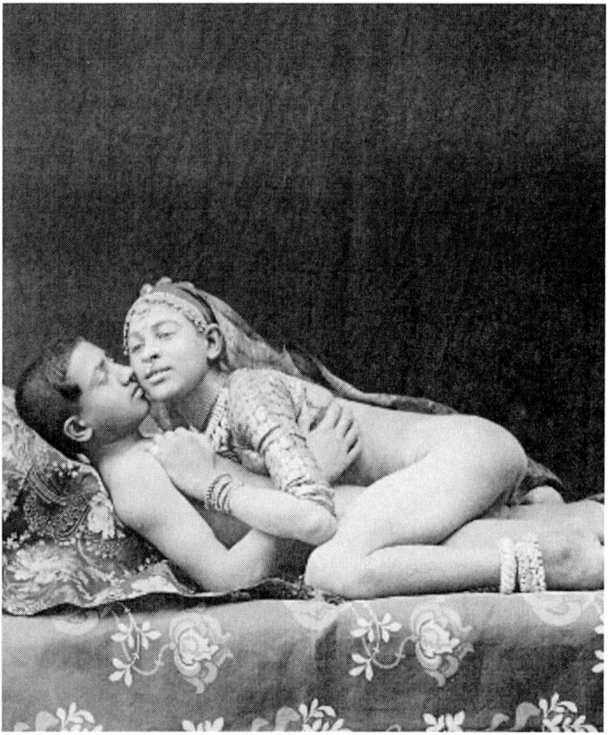

The journey of enjoyment, photo album from the Royal House of Kutch, 1890-1900.

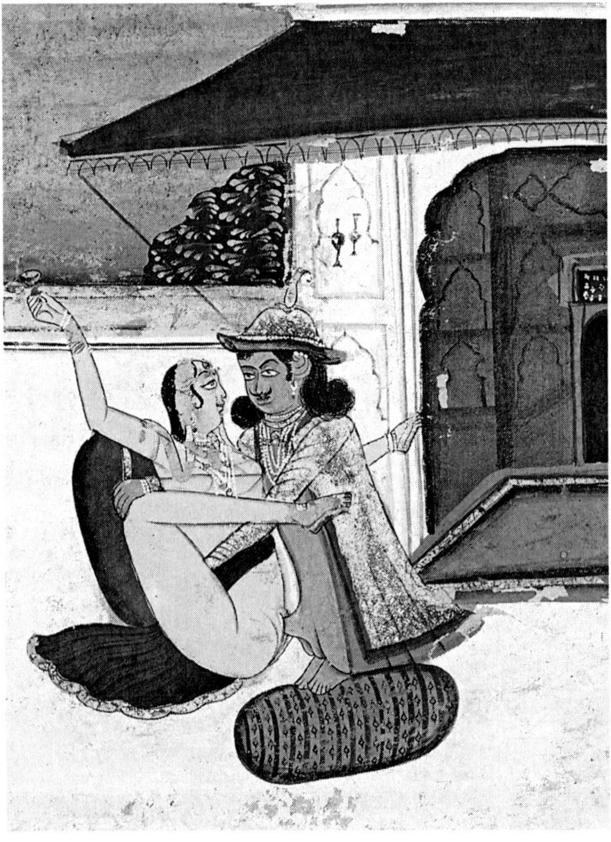

A happy union, Jaipur School, 19th century, natural pigments with gold flange on paper.

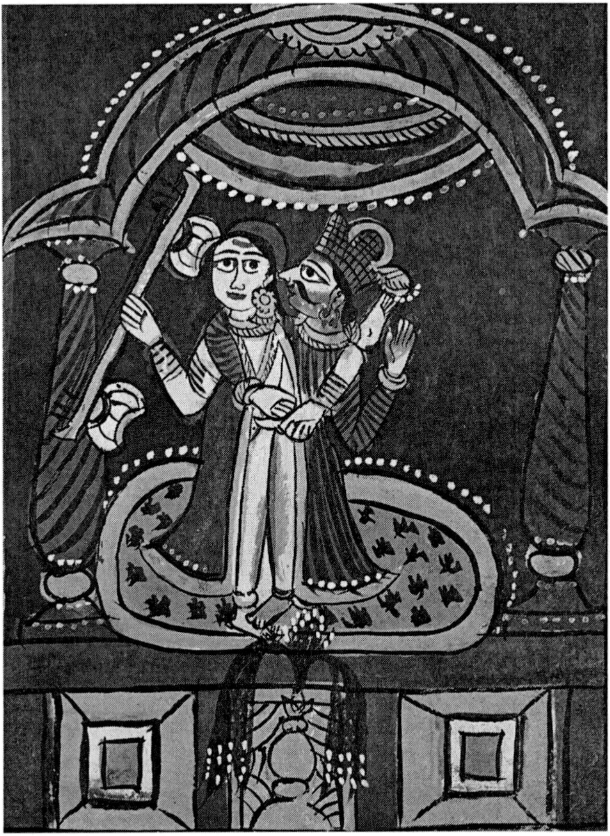

Disrobing the musician, Sirohi School, early 19th century, natural pigments on paper.

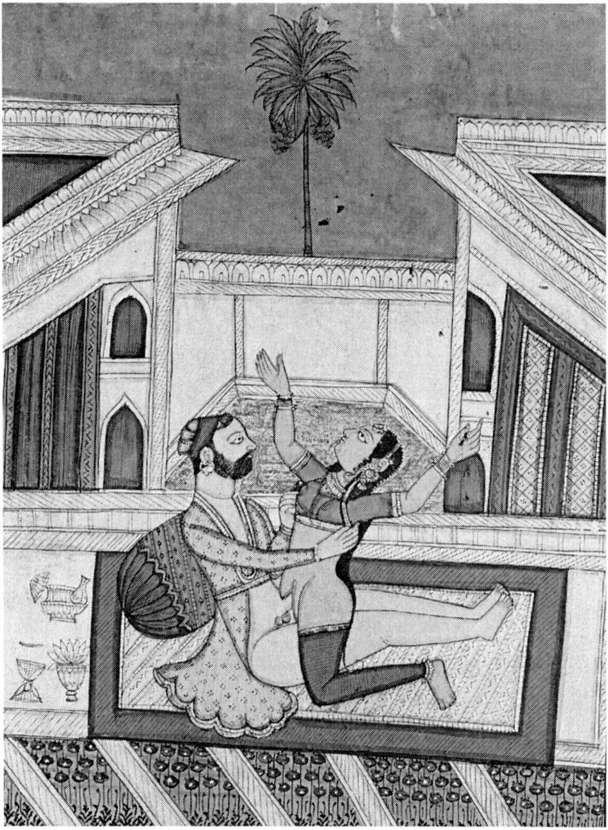

In gay abandon, Orccha School, c. 1800, natural pigments with gold flange on paper.

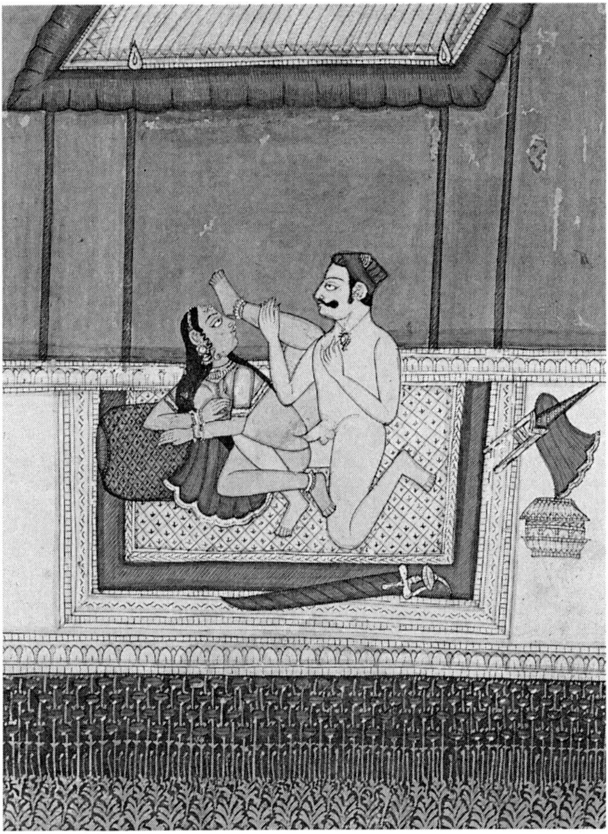

Under the canopy, Orccha school, c. 1800, natural pigments with gold flange on paper.

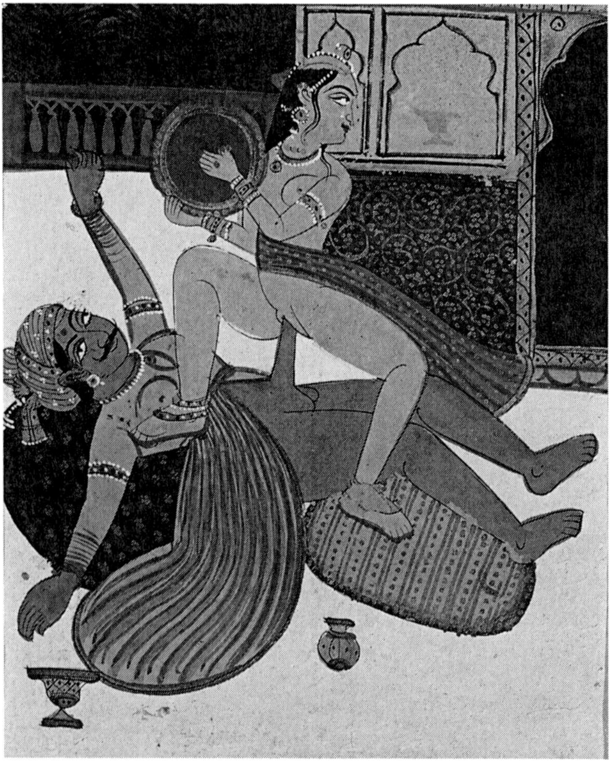

Top: *Wild with joy,* Jaipur School, c. 1780, natural pigments with gold flange on paper.

Opp: *In the boudoir of pleasure,* Nathdwara School, 19th century, natural pigments with gold flange on paper.

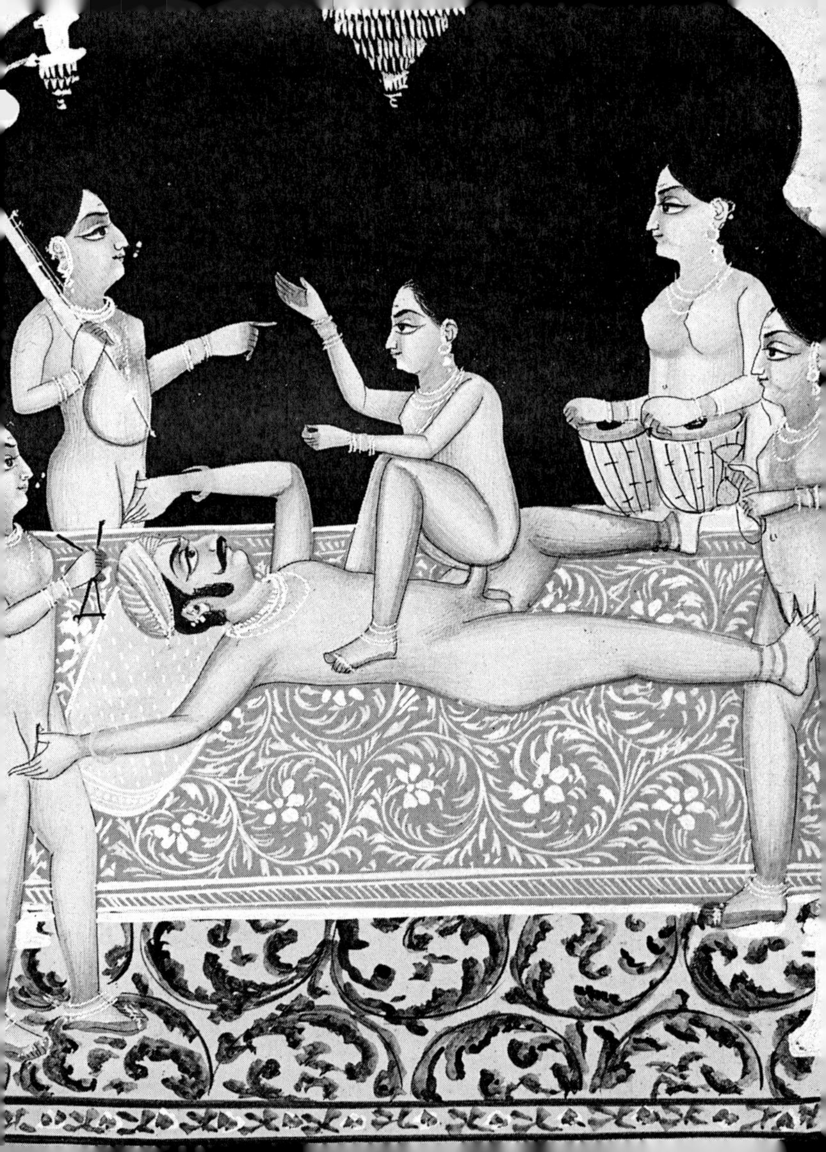

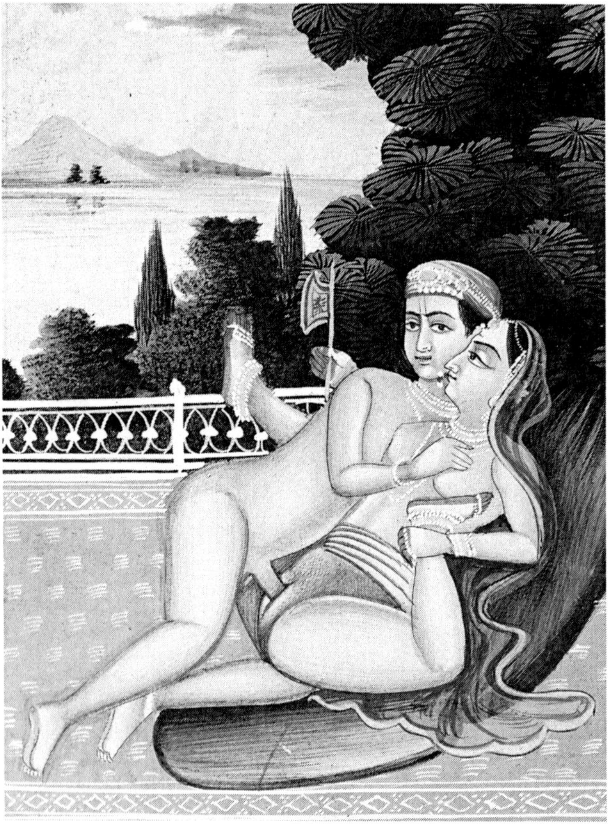

Comfortably close, Nathdwara School, 19th century, natural pigments with gold flange on paper.

Ananda

The concept of *ananda*, or ultimate pleasure, has both the spiritual and the erotic embedded within it. Indian art, literature, and philosophy flourished under the broad canopy of the spiritual. And it is *ananda* which also leads to ultimate bliss, found in heaven, through *moksha*. The other facet of 'heaven' within Indian philosophical and religious thought is similar to a heightened version of a royal palace household. Here, even deities are depicted with erotic attributes. Celestial beings, such as *gandharvas,* possess enormous sexual appetites and the *apsaras* or female celestial beings, too, have pronounced erotic desires and wait in heaven for dead heroes and sages to reward them with superhuman sexual pleasures.

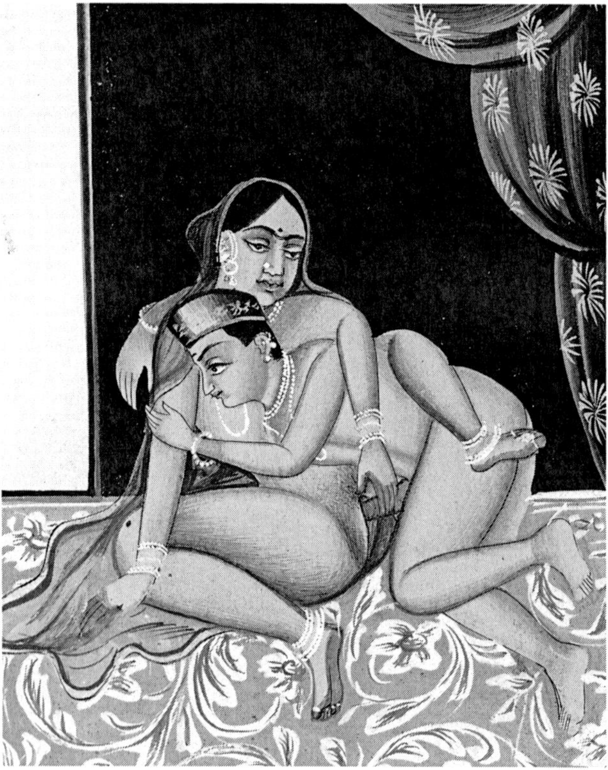

Stolen moments of pleasure, Nathdwara School, 19th century, natural pigments with gold flange on paper.

Opp: *Tender playfulness,* Nathdwara School, 19th century, natural pigments with gold flange on paper.

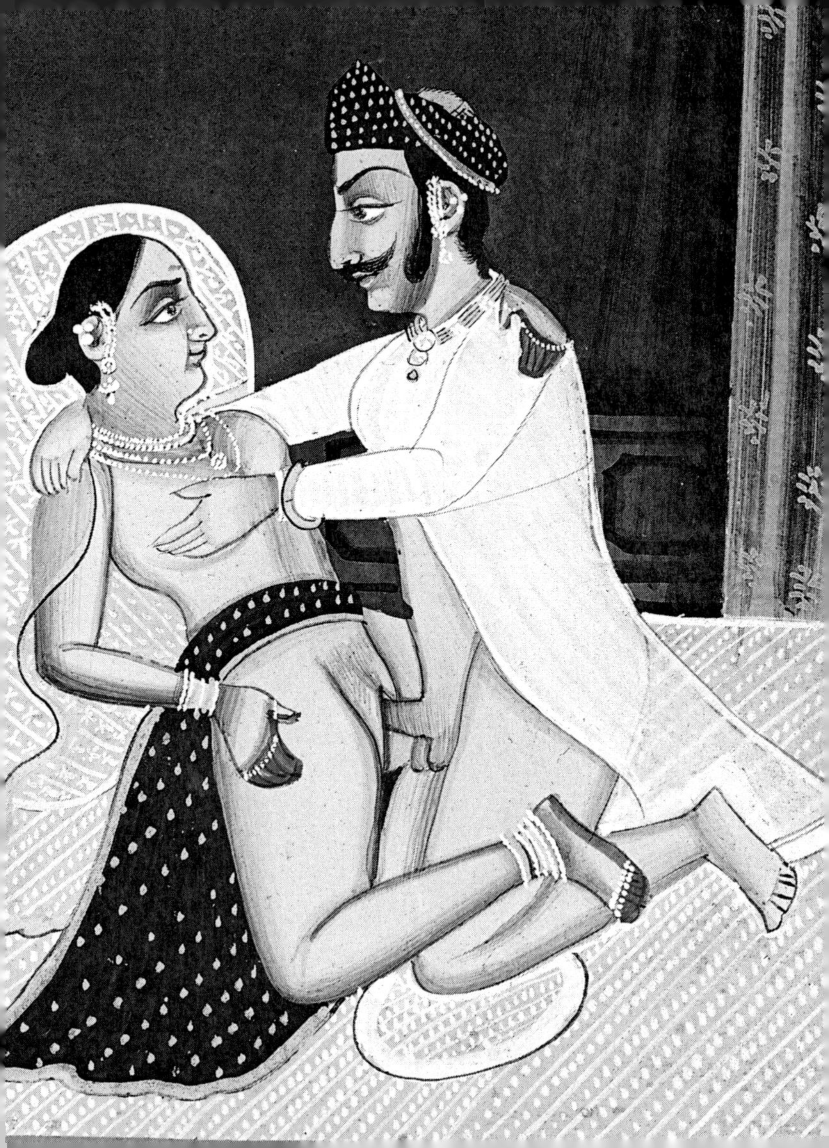

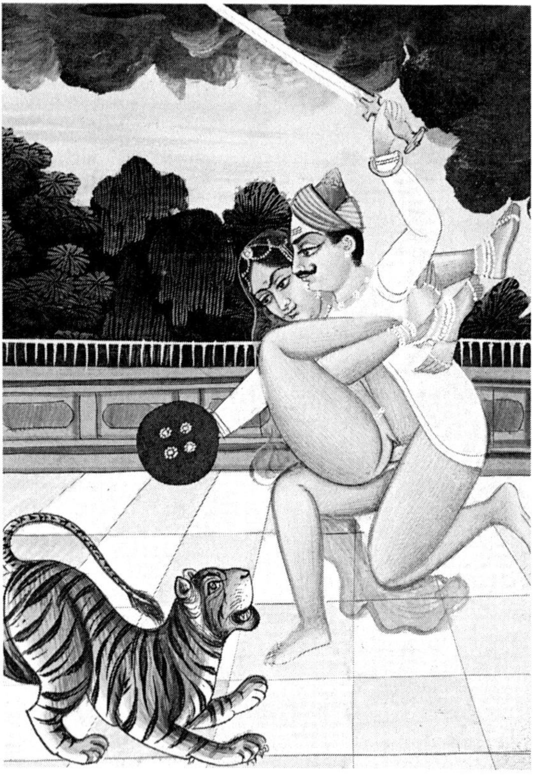

Top: *In defence of love,* Nathdwara School, book with 84 illustrations, 19th century, natural pigments with gold flange on paper.

Opp: *Turning down the heat,* Jodhpur School, 19th century, natural pigments with gold flange on paper.

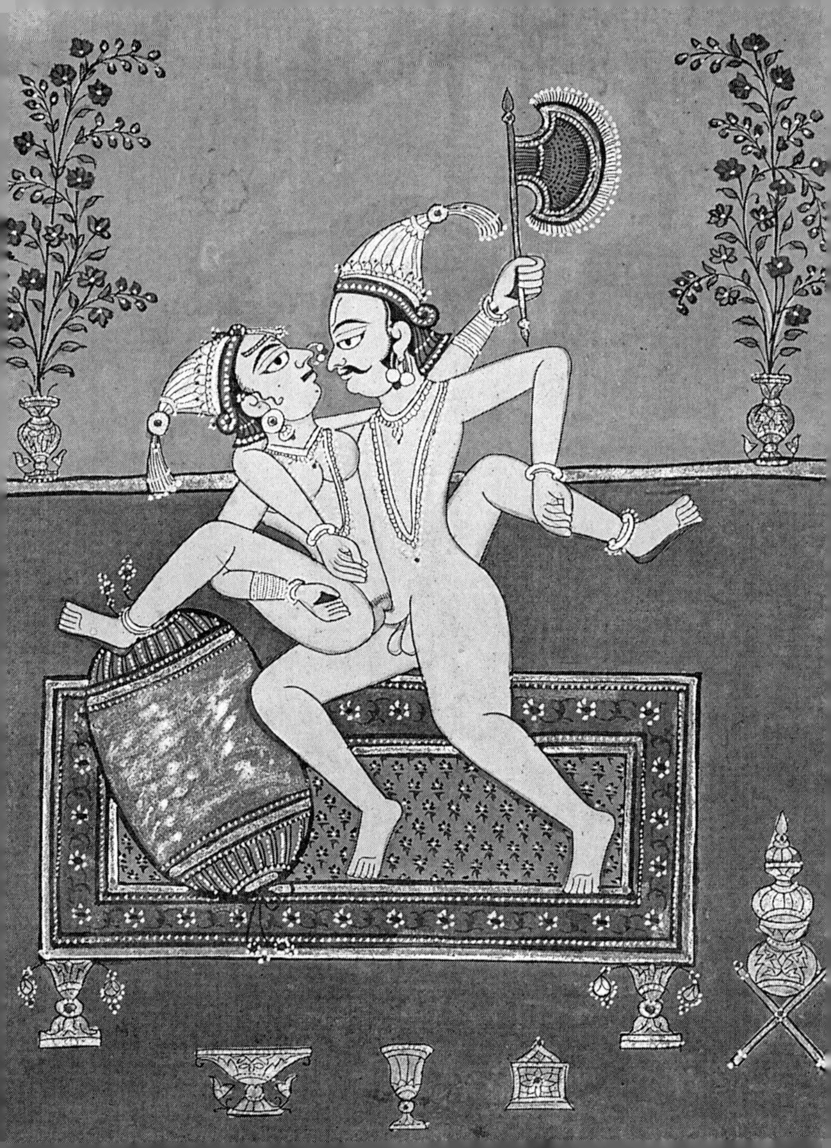

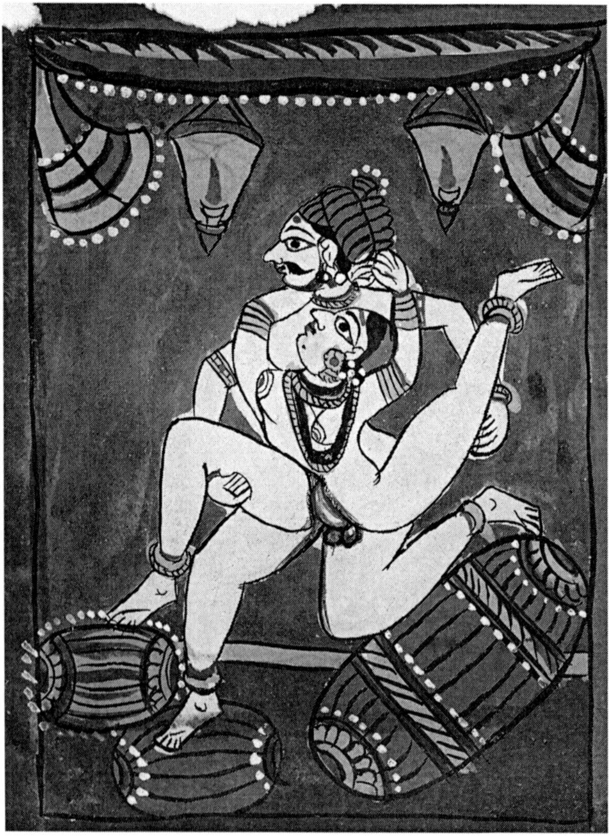

The energetic lovers, Sirohi School, early 19th century, natural pigments on paper.

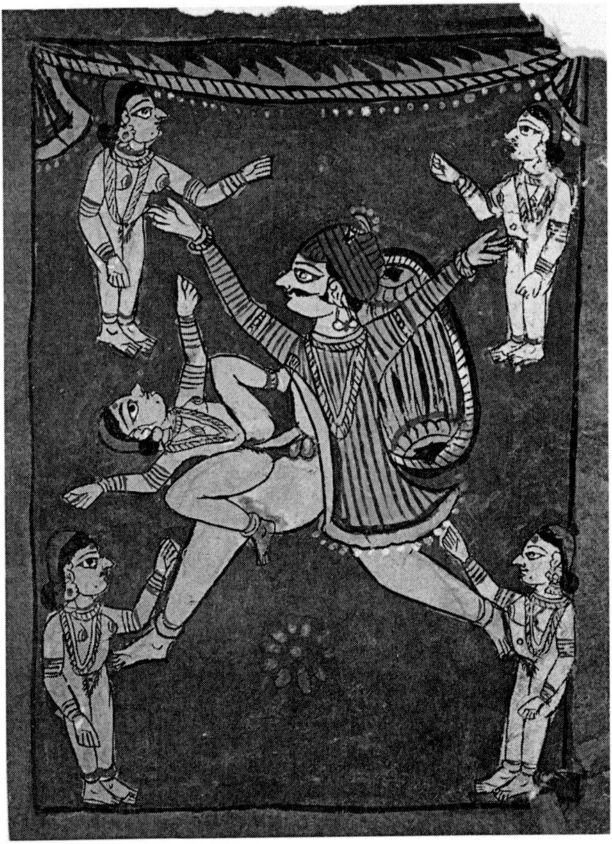

The virile hero, Sirohi School, early 19th century, natural pigments on paper.

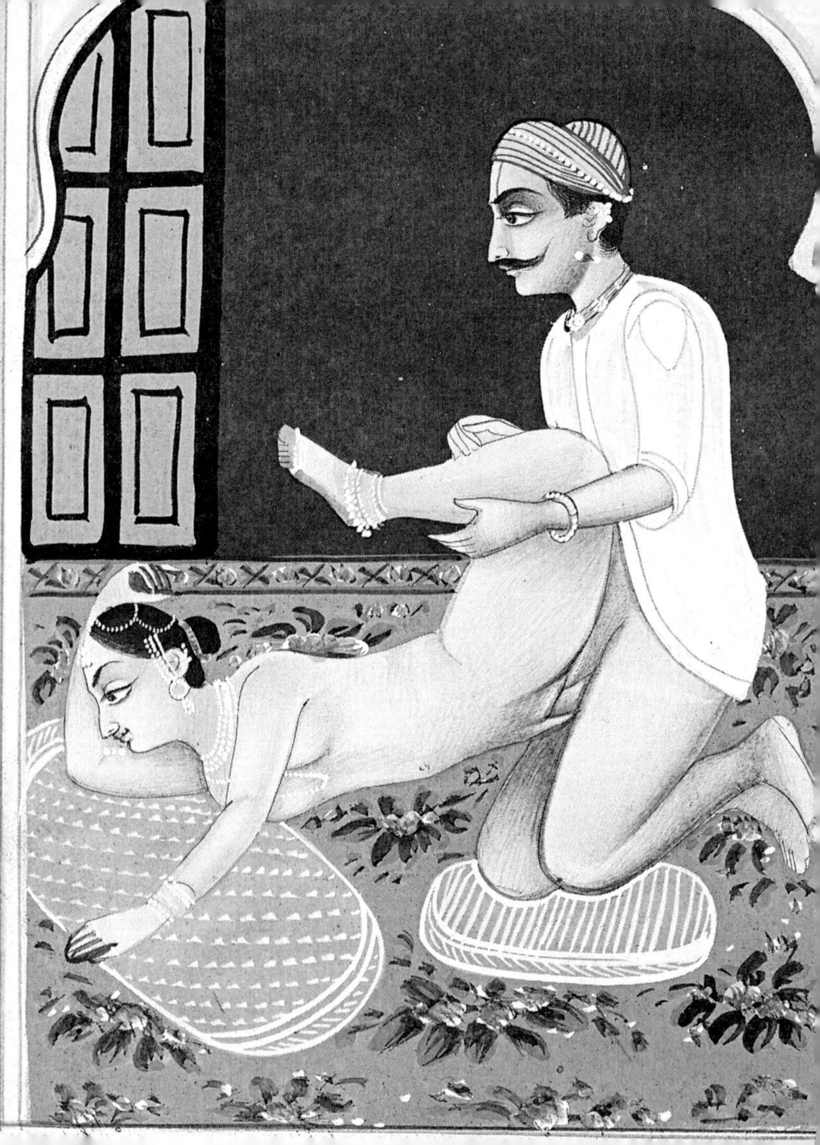

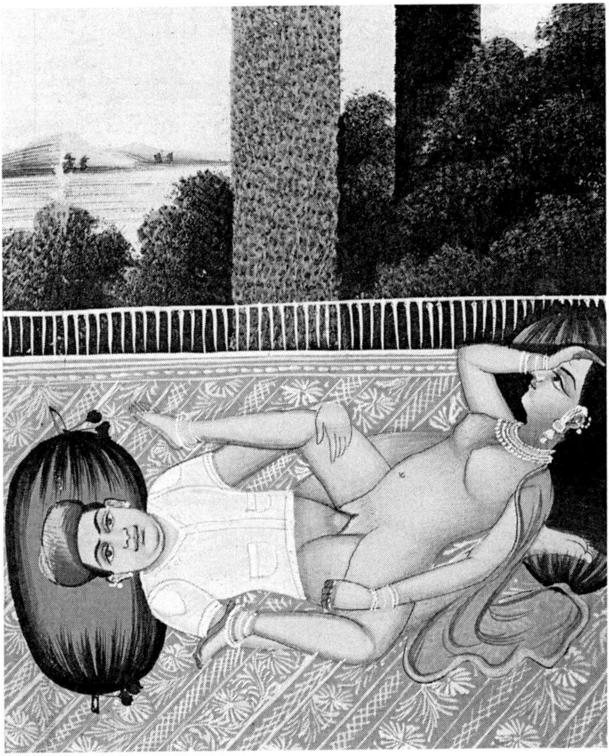

Top: *The gaze of Ananda*, Nathdwara School, 19th century, natural pigments with gold flange on paper.

Opp: *Supple pleasure*, Nathdwara School, 19th century, natural pigments with gold flange on paper.

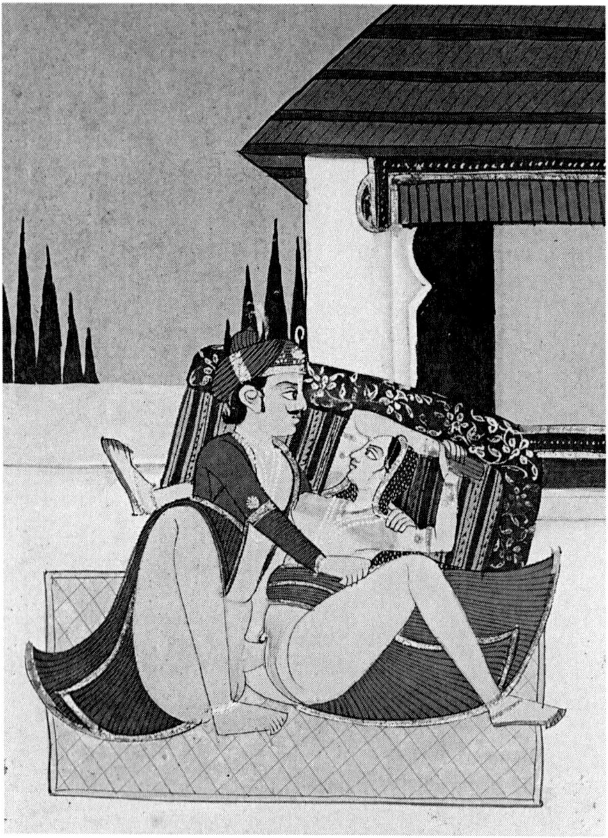

Looking at each other, Jaipur School, c. 1780, natural pigments with gold flange on paper.

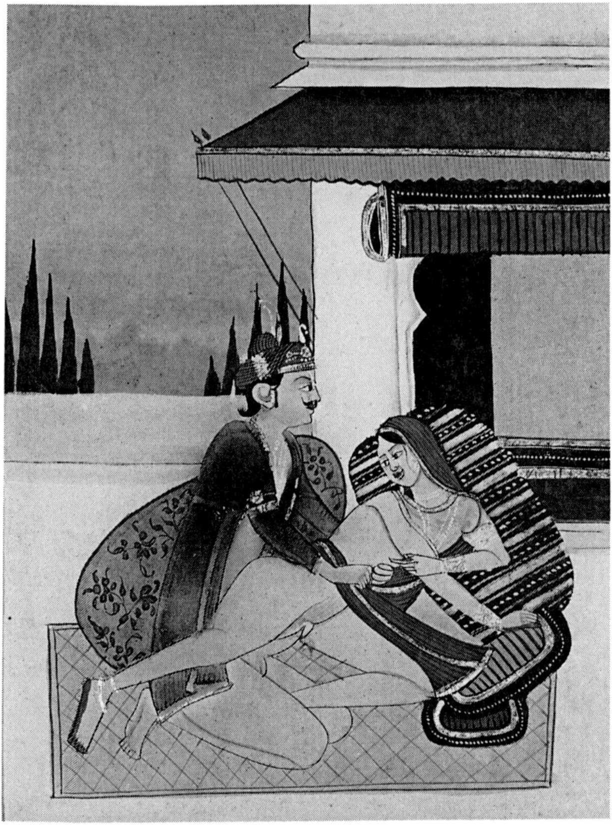

An exchange, Jaipur school, c. 1780, natural pigments with gold flange on paper.

Acknowledgements

All the miniature paintings in the book, and the photographs on pages 22, 23, 42, 43, 56, 57, 60, 61, are from the collection of Anil Relia. I'm grateful to him for granting me and my publisher permission to reproduce them. I'm also grateful to Michel Sabatier for permission to reproduce images of woodcarvings from his collection.

SPEAKING TIGER BOOKS LLP
4381/4 Ansari Road, Daryaganj, New Delhi–110002, India

Book design by Gunjan Ahlawat

ISBN: 978-93-86050-48-9

10 9 8 7 6 5 4 3 2 1

the pocket

KAMASUTRA

a little book of pleasure

Alka Pande

SPEAKING TIGER